# Living
## THE Spiritual
# Principles
## OF Health
## AND Well-Being

Modern science has gone too far in diminishing humankind's spiritual greatness. A new image of consciousness is arising, however, in which the role of love, compassion, and intention —the core of spirituality—is being restored. Science now shows that adherence to a spiritual path is correlated with a longer, healthier life. The bottom line: love heals. This remarkable book shows how.

Larry Dossey, M.D.
Author of *Healing Words* and *The Power of Premonition*

With this book, John-Roger has succeeded in merging the grace of wisdom with the spiritual principles of health, creating what promises to be a seminal work in human consciousness. Everyone who reads this masterpiece gives themselves an experience in healing.

Caroline Myss
Author of *Anatomy of the Spirit* and *Defy Gravity*

A brilliant soulful guide to optimum health on all levels. A must for everyone seeking the truth.

Catharina Hedberg
Co-owner of The Ashram Retreat

# Living
## THE Spiritual
# Principles
## OF Health
## AND Well-Being

# John-Roger, D.S.S.
# with Paul Kaye, D.S.S.

Mandeville Press
Los Angeles, California

## Mandeville Press

P.O. Box 513935
Los Angeles, CA 90051-1935
(323) 737-4055

jrbooks@**mandeville**press.org

www.**mandeville**press.org

Printed in the United States of America

ISBN# 978-1-935492-07-8

Book Design by Shelley Noble

NOTE: *The authors are not medical specialists. This book is
not intended to diagnose, prescribe, or treat. The information
contained herein is in no way considered as a substitute for
care from a duly licensed healthcare professional.*

Everything we think, everything we say, everything we do, is either health creating or health negating. When we begin to look at health and healing that way, we can enter the realm of health creation from anywhere—nutrition, exercise, contemplative practice, or relationship.

*William B. Stewart, M.D.*

Nobody can go back and start a new beginning, but anyone can start today and make a new ending.

*Maria Robinson*

When it comes to eating right and exercising, there is no "I'll start tomorrow." Tomorrow is disease.

*V.L. Allineare*

There are no secrets within you. There is no solution that is hidden from you. There is nothing kept back. All wisdom is available to you at every moment, and it is your challenge and your responsibility to attune yourself to Spirit, and to the God within, so that you may receive the wisdom for yourself.

*John-Roger, D.S.S.*

# CONTENTS

# FOREWORD

I have always known there was more to health and healing than what I learned in medical school. Just prior to embarking on my years of studying to be a physician, the journey was put into a new perspective when a friend gave me some writings about spirituality and health. A few chapters from *The Aquarian Gospel,* a "spiritual" book that was particularly popular at the time, opened my mind to a greater perspective on healing than the narrower focus I was going to learn about in my studies.

When I later dove into the Mind/Body Medicine approach to the patient, I found the distinction between healing and curing both intriguing and profound. A cure is usually seen when an imbalance, or dis-ease, responds to a treatment and can be measured as an objective outcome of resolution. However, there is a greater overarching perspective when healing is present that only the patient can truly appreciate.

A patient may or may not know they have experienced a cure (for example, the treatment of a metabolic disease that is only evident through laboratory testing). However, healing is often a whole-body experience. As it is not measurable like a "cure," the inner experience of healing may even be present when the outer resolution has not occurred. Cancer patients can heal conflicts and imbalances within themselves and their relationships and still go on to die from the cancer, but in a place of peace. Then again, Bernie Siegel writes about cancer patients who have rebalanced through healing and went on to see their cancer resolve into a cure. In *Love, Medicine and Miracles*, Bernie writes, "I do not claim love cures everything, but it can heal and in the process of healing, cures occur also."

In the pages that follow, the reader will be treated to John-Roger and Paul Kaye's multilevel approach to healing. They make it clear that healing occurs on several levels within the person. In my medical practice, I am acutely aware that engaging a patient only on the mental level is not sufficient. That may result in a cure;

however, it may not produce real healing. To inspire change–and therefore healing–I need to engage the part of the person that can shift their awareness to the intrinsic value that being healthier can bring. Sometimes I am better at that than at other times. John-Roger's review of causes and cures provides a usable framework for addressing those deeper issues.

We know 70-80% of the medical complaints that patients present to their physicians have a clear connection to their lifestyle. Choices in activity level, the foods they eat, addictive substances, and high-risk behaviors account for many conditions requiring medical care. But what lies behind those poor choices? What self-destructive thoughts are we running, or are they deeper, unconscious constructs? What family patterns and unhealthy behaviors that we learned growing up do we have to transform so we can truly heal?

This book will assist you in getting to the root of some of these or at least will provide an approach to uncovering many things about yourself relating to the essential causes of your health behaviors. Once your intention is clear and you understand the causes, the steps to rebalancing, healing, and restoring well-being can show up.

Perhaps one of the most simple yet profound ideas John-Roger presents here is an overriding approach that he often suggests: If it works for you, use it, and if it doesn't, let it go. In my experience, there is no place this is more applicable than in health and healing.

Philip Barr, M.D.
*Clinical Director, California Health and Longevity Institute*
*Co-Founder, Conscious Health Consulting, LLC*

# INTRODUCTION

Health is a state of complete physical, mental and social well-being, and not merely the absence of disease or infirmity.

*World Health Organization 1948*

I have written about practical spirituality for over forty years. Over those years science has steadily proven the truth of the words given to me by Spirit. It's now been shown that a positive outlook is good for health; that the mind and emotions directly affect our health; that gratitude is good for health; that forgiveness is good for health; that a loving, caring nature is good for health; and I could name more. In this book I delve more deeply into what I have been saying for years about health and well-being.

I am not prescribing anything for you—that is between you and your physician or health practitioner. My approach and teaching is always a practical one. Any steps you take must keep in mind your individual circumstances. When in doubt, I strongly recommend that you consult with a health professional. What works for one person may not work for someone else.

This book is about taking responsibility for the direction of your health. A guiding principle of this book, and a guiding principle for life, is to use what works for you and let go of what doesn't. Through using the information here and utilizing your inner resources, a clear direction or pathway towards greater health and well-being may emerge. You can then go to your health practitioner and say, "This is what I want to work on."

There are three key physical aspects to health that we all know. We need to feed our bodies with good nutrition, we need adequate, high quality rest, and we need to move our bodies. I look at health and well-being as a multidimensional experience. It involves not only our physical bodies but also the imaginative, emotional, mental, unconscious, and spiritual aspects of ourselves. These dimensions of ourselves will also be explored in this book to see how they can assist us in living a healthy life. To me, the most important aspect is the spiritual dimension in each of us, for that is the part that lives on when the body dies; it is the essence of my work and the context for this book.

This is not a book on dieting or what foods you should eat. There are already hundreds of books on that. Diet is a matter of individual choice, and you should follow the diet that is most compatible with your body and best for your health. Spiritually, it just doesn't make that much difference what you eat, as long as you are not indulging in any addictive patterns. "Success" on the path of Soul Transcendence is much more reflective of the love in your heart than the food that you eat. *(Soul Transcendence is my primary work, see glossary for more details.)*

Similarly, this is not a book about losing weight. You are not the fat you carry, nor are you the guilt you may feel about your weight. Who you are is a beautiful Soul that is always present. So, love yourself unconditionally and know that you are a loving, worthwhile, valuable being, whatever the physical body's expression is at this time.

If you are interested in losing weight, take time to listen to your inner knowing on how to go about it. There are a lot of tools out there that will help you. You have to be willing to activate those tools and to make them work for you. When you reach that point of willingness, pretty much any technique will work, and until you are willing, just love yourself anyway.

Loving yourself no matter what may sound simplistic, but it will work. When you can let go of the frustration, despair, hurt, and judgment you run against yourself, and just love yourself as you are, knowing that your worth, value, and beauty have nothing to do with your physical form, you'll go a long way to releasing the negative energy you've built around you. Then you'll be free to lose the weight, if you choose to.

If you are allowing your physical condition to block you from doing the things that you want to do, you're not being of loving service to yourself. A cornerstone of my teaching is to "Take care of yourself so that you can help take care of others; don't hurt yourself and don't hurt others; and use everything for your upliftment, learning, and growth." You can consider these to be the ground rules for reading this book.

Loving is the most natural way to heal yourself. That means no unreasonable demands or expectations on yourself, and putting your health and well-being into the Light for the highest good. If you get just this, you are on the way to healing and balancing yourself.

The highest teachings express unconditional loving. Unconditional loving is free of judgment, emotions, and dis-ease. As you learn to truly love yourself, your body, the temple of your loving Spirit, will respond in radiant health. However, since you may have spent many years in ways that are less than loving, perhaps you need support and practice. So I recommend you surround yourself with loving people, do loving actions, and participate in those activities that awaken you to the power of loving yourself. In time, as you learn to love yourself (and others), you will create a loving terrain in which your body can heal.

My wish is that this book will be a catalyst and an inspiration for you to put together your own program towards greater health and well-being for the rest of your life. A suggestion—and you could take this as a personal challenge—is that you make one small, significant, meaningful step towards your health and well-being that can be sustained and maintained for the rest of your life. That small step applied consistently can make a world of difference to you.

# The Principles

# Principle 1

# Earn the Trust of Your Basic Self

As a people, we have become obsessed with Health. There is something fundamentally, radically unhealthy about all this. We do not seem to be seeking more exuberance in living as much as staving off failure, putting off dying. We have lost all confidence in the human body.

*Lewis Thomas*

*The basic self's job is to maintain the physical body, to maintain physical functions and all those things that go with it.*

All of us have three selves—the basic self, the conscious self, and the high self. The conscious self is the level that is reading and recognizing the words on this page and understanding them. The level we're communicating on now is called the conscious self because we're conscious of this moment. The conscious self is responsible for making choices and determining the direction you will take.

The high self monitors your overall life plan from a very neutral perspective. When you have feelings of great inspiration, it is more than likely that this is coming from the high self. When you see everything in the world in love, beauty, and harmony, where everything is right and perfect—those moments usually come out of the high self.

The basic self looks after the physical body and is one of the most important and underutilized resources for greater health and well-being. You can relate to the basic self as our animal instinct or the areas of our memory, habits, or emotions. It is good to be aware that the basic self likes habits so it behooves us to learn to work with the basic self more effectively.

The basic self builds the body from the point that the sperm enters the egg. In addition to its key role in the maintenance and health of the body, it is also responsible for the functioning of the psychic centers (chakras) of the body. The basic self is also the center where we hold our habit patterns.

If we want to change something, it is crucial to get the basic self's cooperation. Working with it in love and cooperation is therefore one of the great keys to good health. Our job, as a conscious self, is to give the basic self our loving direction. The basic self's job is to give us the energy to move through the world. It is a beautiful partnership.

Although people who follow a spiritual or religious path often put down or ignore the physical body, in fact it is a fantastic mechanism to work from as you transcend the lower levels of consciousness. It's the only level from which you can experience all levels of the psychic–material worlds and move directly from the physical level into Soul. Therefore it's a good thing to respect the body for the temple that it is.

It is through the basic self that the karma that is to be worked out is brought forward. Karma means action. Most people look upon this as negative, and although it will push you into negative areas, it does so in order that you become aware and gain knowledge of certain patterns and can accomplish in the world.

The basic self does its job very well. If you don't have knowledge of the basic self and how to work with it while walking around in this physical world, your attempting to keep yourself in balance can become a very daunting experience. The more knowledge you can have of the basic self and its job, the more successfully you can function with it and work with it. If you say, "I'm using this body to go through this physical level and I'm using the basic self to maintain physical balance," then you have identified accurately what these levels are, and you will find that you will be able to work with them more freely.

When the basic self is disturbed and can't handle a situation, it wants to have something to do to release its feelings of discomfort. A lot of times, it will want you to eat a great deal. While you have food in your stomach the basic self is working, so it feels better because it is fulfilling its job. Or it may like you to drink or smoke because that gives it something to do and quiets it down. Sometimes it will tap the hands, jiggle the feet, or bite the fingernails—it just wants to be doing something. But for the most part, the basic self wants to complete all the things you've left incomplete. This is a big part of its action. Your job in working with the basic self is cut out for you. *(See Principle #5—Complete)*

*It's important that you work with your basic self in cooperation and love if you want its support.*

It's important that you work with your basic self in cooperation and love if you want its support. If you start berating your basic self, you can produce arthritis, rheumatism, cancer, tuberculosis, and a lot of other diseases. It is so much nicer to say to your basic self, "You did a pretty good job today, and tomorrow we'll do even better."

The way to make the basic self feel good is to love it—not to show affection—to love it. Affection is something you do with your wife or husband or those people who are close to you. We're talking about the love which says, "No matter what you do, I love you." The basic self will be so much easier to work with if you understand that its job is body maintenance, memory, emotions, habits, and releasing karma.

When you look in the mirror in the morning or in the evening, look in your eyes and just say to the basic self, "I love you very much. We're going to work together. It's going to be okay. You keep the energy moving up, and I'll give you good positive direction that will lift us both and help us all."

Sometimes you can contact and connect with the basic self by putting one or both of your hands over the area just above or below the belly button. Sometimes you can gain contact with it by thinking of your pet or an animal you love.

In order to have a good relationship with the basic self, it is absolutely vital that you keep your word with it. If you don't, trust can be lost and communication shut off. The basic self mostly communicates with us in pictures, but you may also get words or intuitive thoughts when contacting the basic self.

If stress is an issue for you, one of the simplest and most effective ways to alleviate it is through belly breathing. This is a simple focus on the rising and falling of your breath, and as you relax and bring the feeling of the breath lower into the belly, it triggers a relaxation response. This process also allows you to more easily get in touch with your basic self and indicates to it that everything is okay.

Breathing more in the chest can trigger a stress response, also known as fight or flight. If you are feeling stressed in your life, get your breath down into the belly, contact the basic self, and let it know that all is well. You'll find it much easier to relax.

The basic self is an integral part of you, and so with everything you do, giving it a form of respect and honor is appropriate. If we're going to have the basic self function with us, we honor it. Honor is a phenomenon of awe. When you see something very, very beautiful, you say, "Wow!" Through awe we honor each other, and we can bring it into us as enthusiasm. With enthusiasm, you honor the basic self as the repository of all good things for you.

A great deal of the time the conscious self works as a mediator between the lower self and the high self. If the feeling comes up, "I'd like to hit you right in the nose"—that's the basic self. The conscious self says, "No, I won't do that." And the high self says, "Love them. That will clear things faster." The high self's approach is more in the area of the lofty ideals.

The basic selves can communicate with each other just as well as the conscious selves do. Our high selves can communicate with one another in a similar way. We are on a great many levels of communication, continually.

Take a moment to give your love and thanks to your basic self. And also give thanks to the conscious self and to the high self. As you give thanks, just move into the fullness and the openness of receiving any healing on any level for your highest good. In fact, one of the most beautiful and gratifying of all prayers is just saying, "Thanks." In reality, that is the only prayer necessary.

When the conscious self asserts its will, it is really quite powerful. But in a showdown of willpower with the basic self, nine times out of ten, the basic self will win. However, when it comes to using the imagination, nine times out of ten, the conscious self will win, because the basic self can only accept what consciousness places in it. So, if you maintain a positive image of completion, the basic self will accept it and work with it. If you place an image forward, the basic sees it and goes to work to make it come about; it asserts energy into those levels to bring it about.

The three selves (high self, conscious self, and basic self) are a perfect marriage. The basic self has the responsibility of maintaining the body, the high self is responsible for holding the spiritual direction, and the conscious self chooses whether or not to go along with the divine game plan. In physical sickness and in health, your high self always holds the spiritual design. If your conscious self rests and gets out of the way, it can permit the basic self to work on healing your physical body.

Try to be aware of the different levels inside you, and get in touch with the basic self to see what a resource it can be to you. Of course, always be loving with it and give it clear direction. Part of that loving is to let it have its say and hear it out in a loving way.

# Principle 2

# Hold the Images in Your Mind That You Want More Of

In my dream, the Angel shrugged and said, "If we fail this time, it will be a failure of imagination."

And then she placed the world gently in the palm of my hand.

Brian Andreas

*Holding the pictures in your mind that you want more of puts the cosmic awareness on notice that you are a force to be reckoned with. And it will start the supply.*

In order to live a healthy, vibrant life, I would be sure to hold pictures in my mind that I want more of. I wouldn't hold other pictures. I just wouldn't do it. That doesn't mean that other images don't come into my awareness; it's just that I don't hold on to them. They come in and they go right on out, and I continue to hold only the pictures that I want.

The basic premise above is repeated over and over again in this chapter. Why the repetition? Because I have been saying this simple idea for years, and it takes awhile for people to get it. It's an approach that won't restrict or hurt you but will expand and amplify you.

To utilize the creative imagination, you take a thought of what you want, losing weight as an example, and you see yourself slimmer. You create that image—you image-in or imagine—and you keep putting that image inside you. You hold that as a focus until you become that.

The key is that you must have the correct image, and when you have it clearly, take that image and put it in your mind and consciousness. You put in what you want more of, what you are going to commit to.

If you're out swimming and you see someone drowning, do you focus on drowning them or do you focus on saving them? Saving them, of course, because they are already drowning. That's exactly the idea I am talking about, and you can apply it for your greater health and well-being.

We are all masters of holding a negative thought or focus and thinking that approach is correct. It's wrong. It doesn't make sense. If you step on a nail, you focus on taking care of the injury, and then you focus on it getting well. Focusing on the pain and it not getting well is not going to help anything. It's very simple, but our ingrained habits tend to pull us towards the negative.

It's been said, "In every day, in every way, I'm getting better and better." But it's only words until you truly see yourself, in your daydreaming or in your imagination, really getting better and better. Then holding the picture in your mind that you want more of becomes a positive use of each day. There is never a dull moment because each moment can be used for your learning, upliftment, and growth.

What we often do with that moment is hold the picture in our mind that we want less of. We hold fear in our mind. We hold worry in our mind. Yet, if we can get a feeling of joy or peace, we can then find a picture to match that in our mind—for example, a puppy or kitten or a lake in the mountains. Then we have a brand new start in this very moment.

It doesn't matter how old your physical body is or whether you're male or female. This joy or peace is not prejudiced at any level. It lets you do as you please, and if that doing has been good, then you'll attract good into you from now on. And if it's been bad, if there is such a thing, you will attract that to you from now on—but you can choose to change. So your big challenge in this world—and it is a big one—is to hold the pictures in your mind that you want more of, not what you want less of, because there is a cosmic law that says "like attracts like."

A vitally important theme in this book is: hold images in your mind that you want more of. I strongly suggest that if you want to go in the direction of better health on all levels, start building that habit now.

When you maintain a positive image, the basic self accepts it and works with it. If you place a clear image forward, the basic self sees it and goes to work to make it come about. Once the basic self has a clear image of the goal, it will work towards it 24 hours a day, even when you aren't thinking about it consciously. The basic self is full of energy to express itself. It works to fulfill those images that it has recorded, even if they're old habit patterns. So, to change a habit, it's a matter of redirecting the basic self to fulfill a new image that is more suitable to you.

How can you heal your body? I'll go back to it again. Keep the pictures in your mind that you want more of. Keep those pictures in your mind and always look towards them. And move your body into those things that you want more of and feel good towards. The alignment between the thought and feeling you have and the moving of the body towards the image starts to heal the body. Let your face light up with the blessing of being alive. Just hold with that image—through everything.

Our subconscious mind communicates with us, and with each other, and does so in picture form. Those things that you want in your life, picture them for your subconscious mind to look at. Make that picture as exact as you possibly can. Remember to always ask that only those things that are for your highest good be brought forward.

Picture the organs of your body that have been disturbing you as perfect. If you've been having trouble with the lower back or a kidney, tell that organ now that it is perfect and perfectly functioning, because that's the way it is designed to be. That's the way it will be—now. It is all now. This second is your eternity. It's brand new.

*When you maintain a positive image, the basic self accepts it and works with it. If you place a clear image forward, the basic self sees it and goes to work to make it come about.*

Imagine your way to vibrant health. We already do a good job of imagining our way to illness. If this process of life is here for us to learn and grow and we can enter into illness, we can reverse the process and enter into health because the path doesn't go one way, it stays open. When we feel like we're stepping out of the Light, we can step right back into it again and go on and keep lifting up into the higher consciousness. The Light and the Spirit are with everyone at all times, regardless. All we are doing is activating it.

The correct use of the imagination is to hold pictures of completion, and to hold the pictures of what we want more of. Truly, a positive outlook by way of visualization takes place on this imagination level. We can therefore choose to see in our creative imagination everyone doing good, everyone being good, everyone having good—and "everyone" includes ourselves! And then, not only will we have it in the imagination, but we will also physically manifest it so that our Light can so shine that it glorifies the God form.

It isn't difficult to do. It is entirely possible for us to picture that possibility in a beautiful way. By not spreading ourselves out too thin, we can let the Light shine in the way it is meant to; in a relaxed, joyful way.

The Bible says, "As a man thinks, in his heart he becomes." And one of the laws of the mind is, "Hold the picture in your mind that you want more of and you'll get it." If you hold the picture in your mind you want less of, you are going to get that. So, when you start getting the things that you don't really care for, and you come complaining to me, I'll say, "Well, what have you been thinking about?" You'll tell me and I'll say, "You see, it works. It's a negative proof, but it is clear proof of how this works."

What do you want more of? If you want more happiness, don't focus upon your despair. Don't focus upon your resentment; that's not happiness. How can you be happy in a hateful situation? Get out of it. If there's nothing you can do, at least don't keep throwing gasoline on the fire around you. It doesn't work to keep hating a hateful situation and expecting it to be good. The concept is to focus upon that which you want more of, not what you want less of. This is because as we focus our mind on negative pictures, the Spirit starts feeding it with subtle energies until that image comes around and captures us. Then we find ourselves going more and more into it until it becomes a functional reality.

Is there anything you can do with the negativity that comes up? Let it go. Is there anything you can do with this thing in your head that keeps you focused on and driving you towards negativity? Get with people who are on an upward path. It's very important to get yourself connected with those people that are going towards health, wealth, and happiness—health in terms of the body, wealth in terms of inner resources, and happiness in terms of the mind.

There is no need to play victim to your mind. You can also transcend the physical boundaries of the mind by focusing upon the transcendent. Instead of focusing upon the boundaries, we focus beyond the boundaries. Instead of focusing upon our lack, we focus upon our supply. You can get out of bed, go to work, or look for a job, and while you're doing all that, breathe in and breathe out and be happy and joyful. Why? Because that's what's really going on.

Hopefully, along the way, you mature and realize you're not part of this—that you're visiting this Earth on vacation and that, really, you are here to go beyond it. At some point in all of this, inside you, the joy that is ever present says, "Hey, I'm Spirit. I am Spirit. My God, I've always been that!" And from that point on, you just focus upon that.

I hope you are getting that the correct use of your creative imagination is one of your biggest keys. I'd like to issue a life challenge for you, and just start out by trying it for a week: hold the pictures in your mind that you want more of, keeping in mind that which is for your highest good.

The challenge for all of us is to hold the pictures in our mind that we want more of. The more details you can get into the picture, the closer you are to getting to the reality of what you're going after. At some point, you'll be able to open your eyes and what you see physically will match the details of the picture that you've held in your mind. Then enjoy it and check out how it works for you.

The imagination level can be looked at in two ways, that's either your nightmare or your creativity. It depends on what you're going to do with it. The power of what is called "positive thinking" is not actually thinking as much as it is holding positive pictures in the imagination of that which you want to come about. What if it's not tangible? What if it's a quality like joy? Then take something and make it a symbol of what you want so you can have fun with it.

*The imagination level can be looked at in two ways, that's either your nightmare or your creativity. It depends on what you're going to do with it.*

The imagination has power over the body, because it's a higher level, and the higher level always rules the lower. That's just the way this thing goes. About two years after a thought has been incubated and seeded in the imagination, it will start manifesting out in the world. "Do I have to wait that long?" In that case, three years for you, because you put a negative thing on top of it with your impatience. You cut off the sunshine to what you planted. "Well, I don't believe you!" Now it's four years.

Some people never get this idea of holding pictures in their mind they want more of. "I never get anything in this world." There you go. You're putting out a lot of "never," so that's what you are getting. If you want health, wealth, and happiness, what does that look like? When you get the image or picture, put it in the Light for the highest good. Hold that image and the thought and feeling that go with it. Then move towards it and Zap! there it is—done.

Don't be stupid. Keep the wonderful things in your mind. Don't keep the moaning, complaining, aggravating type of thoughts. Let them go and replace them with a positive direction. Get some good counseling from somebody who wants to see you have success and is willing to give you the directional information to have the chance of success. Seek them out. Be with those people that are willing to let the Lord shine in them, because they'll help you find the way to your happiness. This is not hard or difficult, but it does take a willingness to let go of the negative and to choose the positive.

If your friends tell you about doom and gloom, tell them you saw the movie last year. It's really as simple as that. If they go on to tell you their horrible experience, just tell them they probably have horrible experiences because that's the way they live their life. Don't let them dump it on you. They won't like it, but then, who needs friends who are carrying garbage around. You can have compassion and be loving, but that doesn't mean that you have to be the dumping ground.

Every image you have in the imagination level becomes real on that level, so we have to learn to only put in motion what we want more of. At the imagination level it happens immediately; however, down here in the physical world, we may never get it, so we have to learn to see it very clearly in our mind. In other words, we get a goal. Then we keep the mind on the goal while taking the necessary small steps, in a relaxed way, to get it. We also get the emotions enthusiastic about the goal, and we then just walk the body through the process.

So I hope you are getting this. Don't hold the pictures that you want less of because this planet already has a lot of negativity in it—negative in terms of a battery. The Soul is the positive polarity, while the imagination, mind, emotions, unconscious, and the physical body make up the negative polarity. That's five negatives to one positive, but it functions like twenty-five negatives to one positive. That's why we can't allow ourselves the luxury of a negative thought. Does that become a little more apparent to you? When you enter into rampant negativity, you're killing yourself. You have made the negativity something much, much larger than you think you are. But you are Soul. Get with the program.

Here's the neat thing. There's a sixty second "Cancel" button for thoughts you don't want in your mind. You just say, "Cancel" or "Deflect." What it boils down to is, the choice has always been yours, it always will be yours, and all that heaviness you go through is your choice. If you don't like that choice, change the choice by activating your consciousness in the path that will provide for you what you want, not by leaping out there, wishing for it, but by a methodical, step-by-step progression.

# Principle 3

# Eliminate and Detoxify

The body is reasonably resilient. However, if you have indulged too much, help your body to recover in the simplest way. Get plenty of fresh air and exercise. Flush your system through with plenty of water. You don't need expensive remedies for getting back from somewhere you should not have been in the first place. Try not to go there again.

*Dr. Derek Lohman*

*Disease isn't what we take in— it's what we don't eliminate.*

*What we do not eliminate is what makes us sick.*

A major part of this book is to look at the cost-free and under-utilized resources that we have available to improve our health and well-being. The reality is that we're the most medically dependent generation ever and, as we read in the news just about every week, obesity and hypertension (along with many other health concerns) are pandemic. We all know from experience that health maintenance can be very expensive, but by intelligently using our own inner resources along with the extensive free information that is available to us through the Internet and other sources, we can reduce those expenses and move ourselves in a positive direction towards health and well-being.

For example, something as simple as eating less volume of food, but more nutritious food, can go a long way to improving our health. Walking three times a week for 20–30 minutes also can have a significant impact on the health of the body and on the mind and emotions as well. And the positive health effects from simply relaxing and reducing the amount of self-induced stress are well documented.

Elimination and detoxification are essential aspects of maintaining a healthy life. The two phrases on the title page of this chapter are important to absorb as you go about learning and applying this principle: Disease is not what we take in; it's what we don't eliminate, and what we do not eliminate is what makes us sick. Essentially, we need to let go of what no longer serves us.

Let's look at detoxification from a multidimensional perspective.

*Physical Detoxification:* This is where we let go by resting and relaxing the body. So much detoxification takes place when we sleep, so adequate sleep is very important for health. Eating less and more healthily will also detoxify the body, as will fasting. Movement is very important in detoxifying the body, whether it's active movement through walking or yoga or passive movement through massage.

*Emotional Detoxification:* This is where we let go of our attachments and positions, which give rise to emotions of fear, anger, etc. One of the easiest and best ways to let go is through forgiveness.

*Mental Detoxification:* This is where we let go of the judgments we have held against ourselves, others, events, and circumstances. Forgiveness, once again, is the big key to letting go of judgments.

*Unconscious Detoxification:* This is where we clear unconscious blocks to health in the body. A very effective technique for doing this is free-form writing. *(See a complete explanation of free-form writing in the appendix.)*

*Spiritual Purification:* This is letting go and letting God. We can do this very effectively through meditation and most effectively through spiritual exercises. *(See an explanation of spiritual exercises in the appendix.)*

Two of the greatest healing mechanisms on this planet today are breathing and fasting. Breathing increases the heart rate, opens the pores of the skin, and increases the metabolism. The very act of exhaling is a detoxification mechanism. Even if your physical condition does not allow you to fully fast, taking less food into your system or eating less of foods that are unhealthy for you will allow the body to detoxify.

We live or die at the cell level, and since our tissues and organs are made of cells, it's important that those cells get oxygen, get good nutrition, and eliminate what is no longer needed.

I have come up with two important laws dealing with health:

1) The living body is designed to function in the direction of health, and sickness is the effect of obstructing natural function.

2) Sickness is the result of the body's struggle to eliminate internal toxins resulting from a bad environment and bad habits.

The negative judgments we make create negativity in the consciousness. That negativity can be looked at as an internal poison. If we are sick physically, we often need to go to the next higher or more subtle level to invoke the healing. For example, we can go to the imagination where we can envision our body healing and hold the image of wellness. If our problem is an emotional one, we can go to the mental level and perhaps change a belief we have or change our thinking to a more positive frequency by, for example, thinking happy thoughts. Going to the next level above where we are is a useful tool to keep in mind as we move towards wellness. It's when we are sick and we do not change, that we create disease. That can often be our bad habits taking control and running us.

Elimination takes place at lots of levels. The five fundamental ways we do that in our body are: our lungs through breathing, our kidneys through our urine, our bowels through our stool, our skin through sweating, and our tongue which we can cleanse by scraping it in the morning.

Of the above, the easiest way to eliminate is to breathe, ideally, the cleanest and most oxygen-rich air you can find. The ocean is a wonderful place to go if you have access to it. Another essential form of elimination is sweating. You can encourage it actively, by exercising and moving the body, or passively, by sweating in a sauna or bath. Drinking pure water is a marvelous way to flush out toxins and assists the kidneys in their function.

You'll be glad to know that there is a simple way to detoxify that applies to all levels. The easiest way we can eliminate disturbances and detoxify is through loving ourselves and others. Loving it all is the best way.

Upon arising in the morning when the system is relatively empty and before eating anything, you can drink a glass of pure water. If you wish, you can build up slowly to drink one-half liter and then a full liter. Listen to your body to see what works for you. It's best to drink the water all at once. This practice is an ancient one and really assists the body to flush out toxins.

Although this practice may hydrate the body, its main purpose is to flush the system. Hydration is best achieved by drinking small amounts of water frequently throughout the day. By the end of the day, you'll have drunk a lot of water without the need to urinate often, and you'll likely feel good and refreshed. Hydration is vital for the body as so much of the body's composition (about 60%) is made up of water. It's one of the simplest, yet neglected, things we can do for our health.

If not eliminated, environmental toxins in the body will go into our extracellular fat and into the connective tissue that lies around, in, and between the tissues. The more fat we have increases our capacity to retain more toxicity. Exercise will start dumping the toxicity from the fat into the tissue and will flush it out through perspiration, urine, the breath, and our bowel movements. If we're constipated, we are retaining toxins in our system, and that's not healthy for us.

I can't emphasize enough the importance of effective breathing. It affects everything we do. It assists with reducing our stress levels, elevating our state of mind, improving the health of our bodies, and amplifying our spiritual attunement. Keep in mind this principle: it's not what you are eating that's killing you; it's what you're not getting rid of that's killing you, and one of the most effective elimination systems is exhalation.

When we think of breathing, we often say, "Take in a deep breath." But perhaps we should say, "Exhale. Now receive in a breath." The exhalation is really the key to correct breathing technique as it opens the space for the oxygen to be received. These days, with less oxygen being available to us in the air (particularly if we live in the city), it makes sense that if we have a more effective and efficient breathing mechanism we can get more oxygen into our lungs and we can be healthier.

If you have an imbalance, restriction, limitation, or illness, it can be very helpful to identify the belief system or the emotion or thought or judgment that is connected with it. Identifying and naming it can allow our consciousness to then let it go. You can work with the basic self to identify the patterns that are blocking you. *(See 30–Day Health Program for assisting you to identify patterns to work with.)*

Here is a very brief five-point plan of health. All are very key points:

1. *Move your body—stretch, take a walk.*

2. *Drink sufficient water—good water—to keep the system flushed.*

3. *Watch that you don't flood your emotional body with hormones from the glandular system. (This is covered in more depth in* Applying the Principles: Less Stress)

4. *Watch your thinking so that you create a system of self-talking that talks you into greater vitality and health.*

5. *Keep the images in your mind that you want more of.*

Our bodies adapt and then adopt a new way of being. If you have a habit of negative thinking, the body will then adapt to it and, at some point, adopt it to a new habit pattern that works against our health. When we have adopted a new way of being that is not health-producing, disease can appear. We may go to the doctor, but the medication may not be enough. Yes, the symptoms may go away and we'll feel a measure of relief, but the consciousness that produced the illness is still there.

*If you have an imbalance, restriction, limitation, or illness, it can be very helpful to identify the belief system or the emotion or thought or judgment that is connected with it. Identifying it, naming it, can allow our consciousness to then let it go.*

For example, someone with asthma may use a bronchial inhaler to relieve their symptoms. Then they also may cut down on their milk and sugar intake so they don't have as much mucus and the bronchioles are able to function more freely. However, if they haven't cleared the pattern that caused the asthma in the first place, it can show up somewhere else in the body—and not necessarily in the pulmonary system. It could show up in the skin, it could show up in the liver, it could show up anywhere there is an inherited weakness. As the person gets older, the pattern, combined with their weaknesses and genetic predispositions, becomes the illnesses and diseases that they really don't want. It's far better to stop the negative thinking, or the emotional flooding, or the bad habit, before they get to that place.

A simple way to detoxify the system is fasting. Of course, check with your health practitioner before doing this since the effects and benefits will differ with each individual. However, fasting does not have to be long or complicated. Even fasting over a 24 hour period, from noon to noon can be very helpful. If you are going to attempt a fast, make sure you have at least one bowel movement a day. It's critical.

Another approach that has been found to be very effective is to stop eating after 7:30 p.m. and not eat again until breakfast at 7:30 a.m. You will have effectively fasted for 12 hours. If you do this on a regular basis, you will be giving your body a much–needed rest and an opportunity to "take out the trash" without being disturbed. Again, check with your health practitioner before doing this.

Reducing your food intake will start to detoxify the body. When attempting any form of detoxification, make sure to increase the amount of water you drink because you want to keep your system flushed as the body lets go of toxins.

When you begin to eat less, the body, instead of using the food to feed the disease, allows the disease to surface and come out, and you can actually get sicker than you were before. But when the disease leaves, it's such a good feeling that some people want to take the fasting to the next level, called death. So it's really important to undertake a cleanse under the supervision of a health practitioner who is monitoring with you.

Most diseases aren't because we're fat or thin, but are because of the vibration level we hold inside of us. Food feeds the vibration. We live on the vibration that goes from the food into the body. Food as a substance is poison to the body. Food as an essence is life. Food is energy; food is our natural medicine. If we don't eat, we die. It is a source of life so, ideally, we should get the essence out of food without putting the bulk in.

*Keep in mind that detoxification can be letting go on lots of levels. Forgiveness could be a detoxification program for you as you let go of judgments from your consciousness.*

We can be looked at as a walking sewage tank (not an image to hold in our mind but for educational purposes). The faster we can get the sewage out of us, the better off we are. So moderation in eating, instead of overeating, is a healthier approach. It's also financially healthier because you don't have to buy a lot of food that is not good for you. This then translates to your not spending money on things that you really don't need in order to cover the lack you may be feeling. You're not burdening yourself down; you are letting go.

It can be very helpful to follow the old adage: Breakfast like a king, lunch like a prince, and dine like a pauper. Time and time again in health literature, both conventional and alternative, it is said that breakfast is the most important meal of the day. It is not healthy to forego breakfast and lunch and then have a massive dinner, because not having any fuel (in the form of food) during the day will cause your body to pull energy from the adrenal glands and other glands of the endocrine system in order to maintain its functioning. Over time, the glands get exhausted.

Keep in mind that detoxification can be letting go on lots of levels. Forgiveness could be a detoxification program for you as you let go of judgments from your consciousness. You could choose to go on a mental fast—creating fewer negative thoughts and keeping your mind focused on the positive. Or you can go on an emotional fast of less worry. There are a lot of creative ways to approach this. The important thing to understand is that holding on to garbage, on any level, does not serve you.

# Principle 4

# Relax

*So what can we do to have better health?*

*Be patient and relax.*

*If we honest-to-God could understand hat concept of being patient and letting the body relax, illness would vacate.*

The transition from tenseness and worry, to equanimity, receptivity, and peace, is the most wonderful of all those changes of the personal center of energy. And the chief wonder of it is that it so often comes about, not by doing, but by simply relaxing and throwing the burden down.

*William James*

Tension is who you think you should be. Relaxation is who you are.

*Chinese Proverb*

To let go and let God is to relax and be patient. What if, right now, God is using you to bring His Light and power into this physical-level world? What if, right now, you are living in accordance with God's plan for you? What if your feeling a little sad and lonely is a tool for you to know yourself more deeply? What if the house burning down is a way God has designed to release you from a lot of worldly attachments and lift your attention to His presence? What if all things here are designed for your greatest growth and upliftment? If you can catch that vision, it will be easier for you to let go and let God.

You cannot get away from the essence of Spirit within you. If you try to deny that essence, the result is disturbance and imbalance. The butterflies in your stomach are you placing yourself against yourself. You don't need to do that. You only need to relax, to let go, and to allow the ongoing process of Spirit to take care of you. Not a single moment goes by that does not bring you the opportunity to know the Soul more deeply and more fully. You are the vehicle for experiencing and knowing your Soul. So relax, hold back nothing, and let your Soul be. When you make space for the blessings of Soul to manifest, you become a living blessing.

Give yourself time to let your life unfold within God's timing and in God's way. Trust the Spirit. Let Spirit do for you what you may not have the wit to do for yourself. God takes perfect care of you, if you will only allow it. Life can be very exciting when you let go and let God, when you relax and are patient. If you push for your way, you can end up with difficulty. If you flow with God's will, you're free.

The Spirit is everywhere. So when you relax a position and let it go, the Spirit, the Light, will fill that space. And when you are attuned to Spirit and are experiencing the love of Spirit, the negativity of others does not matter, and your own negativity does not matter. There is love and forgiveness for everything and everyone.

Our bodies build their form around the energy we place out. If we misuse our energy by putting our attention in the wrong place, the body will build its form around it. For example, if you worry a lot, it will be reflected in your tense shoulders and your tight stomach. When we start to use our energy correctly, our shoulders loosen, the stomach relaxes, the energy starts moving into the areas that have been blocked or closed off, and the body starts aligning itself spontaneously. Correct use of energy makes everything liquid, relaxed, and smooth. The body will line itself up and re-form itself according to your conscious thought and pattern of behavior.

The lesson for us here is that if we don't change our behavior, the body will go back to its previous condition. If we are willing to listen and watch, we'll find that the body is not only educating us in how to get well but also showing us how to change the condition that produced the imbalance or illness.

When we are tense, we hold on to what isn't there. We tend to fight and resist as a way of showing strength. Living this way is more a sign of weakness. Relaxing and letting go demonstrate true strength.

When you are relaxed, you are more sensitive and aware. You know not to react when someone says something potentially upsetting or negative. You have the presence to say inside you one very effective word, "deflect." This single word can work wonders against a verbal or psychic attack. There is no need to give up your center for someone else's upset or let negativity build in or around you. It can be handled in a relaxed way.

*The best course is to stay in your loving. There is absolutely no need to play the game that you are no good or that you are not worthy. It's a fool's game. Claim that you are divine and allow yourself to soar in that awareness.*

If someone pushes against you physically, emotionally, or mentally, yield and let go. Don't be there. Be on the other side of them. Be like a revolving door—one door gives as you push, the other follows behind. In this way, you preserve the quality of relaxation. If you find yourself starting to be stubborn or resistant, it's better to give up your position than lose the quality of relaxation and centeredness in order to preserve that position.

The basic principle of letting go, of relaxation, will produce a softness and kindness in your demeanor. Others will often mistake that kindness for weakness. So be light-hearted, good humored, and let there be vitality in your relaxation. Resistance, like tension, is just opposing something that, in reality, is not there. You may feel justified in your opposition, but it is really a strike against yourself. When you get right down to the core of it, we are only upset with ourselves.

The best course is to stay in your loving. There is absolutely no need to play the game that you are no good or that you are not worthy. It's a fool's game. Claim that you are divine and allow yourself to soar in that awareness. Do not fear who you are. Relax into your very cells and know you have everything you need in this moment.

When you feel tension, let go of your resistance. When you feel life is too hard, stop pushing. When you stop the push, you may feel less tired. Are you pushing to get hold of something that is not yours and never will be?

If you can stop for a moment in your thinking and your questing and listen to the silence, you may start becoming aware of many levels of consciousness, and of the fact that you are a multi-dimensional being existing on all levels simultaneously. The trick is to learn to shift your awareness to where you wish to be.

It isn't life's events that cause stress, but it is our reaction to those events that activates the symptoms of stress. For the most part, stress is internally generated by our negative attitude towards ourselves and what is going on in life. The choice of our attitude, choosing between being tense or relaxed in a situation, can be made at any moment. You may thrive on the thrill of stress, but it is likely that there is an addiction to the surge of adrenaline. With practice you'll find that being completely present with whatever is going on is far more thrilling.

We lose nothing by slowing down. That moment of quiet—or nothingness—of silence, is when we find out that, inwardly, we are wealthy beyond measure. We're no longer hung up, but we're free and flowing, and we joyously realize that, despite momentary appearances to the contrary, things have been moving our way all along.

It's important to relax because you can never win with resistance. You win when you approach each situation you meet by slowly expanding your energy field—reaching out to meet and encompass it.

So why not go a little slower in your life? Take a little more care with everything around you. Practice a little patience, because tension and fear create the blocks that stop the flow of life through you. As you take each situation as it comes, one at a time, it's very easy. As soon as you feel overwhelmed or reactive, relax, rest, and gently pull your energy field back in, strengthening it by being still. That moment where you observe and do nothing moves you back into your center, into Spirit and Soul.

Relax. Don't grab. Grabbing is tension. You can't truly possess or hold onto anything anyway. All you can do is utilize what's in front of you. If you try to possess, you lose. You can't even possess your own body. But if you love yourself, if you love the Soul within, you have access to all things. When you realize that God has produced all things for your upliftment, learning, and growth, you start relaxing automatically.

When you want to manipulate someone or something it indicates that you haven't found the spiritual place within where you exist as the Beloved. The one who has "got it" could care less about manipulating anything because they see the total picture of how everything has its timing and is right on schedule. So they sit back in a very relaxed state. Spirit pours through them and brings to them everything they need, and people say that they lead a charmed life. No, they lead a very relaxed life. They don't get irritated or upset by things.

It's really a nice day when you can sit by yourself and not have any problems. That's rest. You let go and a smile comes over your face knowing that you were the source of your problems, and all the people you blamed as being your problem were only reflecting to you your state of imbalance.

When we hold on to materiality, we find that the materiality is really holding us. Yet, when we relax, we open to an expansive place where anything can happen, where there are so many possibilities. Many of us are unwilling to go to that place. We want a guarantee that everything will be okay, that we'll have enough money for the rest of our lives. Since that approach is not the place of openness or spontaneity in which the Spirit resides, we automatically withdraw from the immediacy and intimacy of life. We freeze and become tense. We move into resistance, and thus we build our prison and live in lack.

This past habitual activity stays within our cell structure, in various parts of our body, and creates pressure within us. One way to handle this is to just keep telling ourselves to relax in order to let our muscle, nerve, and fascia structures be healed. This can be a verbal comment that you make to your mind, and you may have to actually lie down and cover your eyes so that the cells begin to quiet.

You can touch your face as a cue that when you tell yourself to relax, all the muscles in and around your eyes and the parts of your body that you designate will relax wherever you are touching them. I would tell myself that whenever I do that, it will relax the muscles. Then I would take it a step further and say to myself that every time I think of relaxing through my touch, the muscles, nerves, and fascia will automatically start to release unnecessary pressure and tension and relax.

*So why not go a little slower in your life? Take a little more care with everything around you. Practice a little patience, because tension and fear create the blocks that stop the flow of life through you.*

Then I would bring this to a point where every time a designated area of my body, let's say my shoulders, get tight, it will automatically trigger a relaxation response. So no matter what situation comes up, as soon as the shoulders tense, relaxation is immediately triggered and they let go. It may take you awhile to have that response, as it takes practice to reach the point where, in the moment of stress, you just relax and let things flow the way they want to, but it is well worth taking the time to practice.

If your day is busy and you need more energy than what you've woken up with, you can take a quick nap to revitalize yourself. If you are on the go and you need an energy boost, you can also take a moment with yourself to be quiet and to relax a single muscle. Energy is then released out of the tightness and is available for your use, and you are now ready to go again. I've also trained myself that when I touch my two fingers together in a certain way, I immediately go into a deep, inner relaxation that rejuvenates me.

So, whether it be in your work, your play, or your spiritual activities, one of the most important qualities you can bring into your life, in activity or at rest, is relaxation. It is the simplest way to regenerate your energy and move your body into greater health and well-being.

# Principle 5

# Complete

*One of the most useful things I can say to you for living in this world is, if you want to have greater health and more energy, move things towards completion.*

Nothing is so fatiguing as the eternal hanging on of an uncompleted task.

*William James*

In life, satisfaction is experienced when activities are brought to a state of completion. Loss of energy and loss of control are functions of incompletion. The result of completing things releases one's ability to create.

*William A. Ward*

This life is very easy. Do and complete, do and complete, do and complete—no karma. On the other hand, just say you're going to do and then not do–karma. Start to do and then not finish—more karma. Feel bad about all that—more karma. It's obvious we've got more karma than we've got completion.

This whole world boils down to one word, energy. That energy is either used for you or used against you, but it is used. It's extremely exciting to know because the more you can complete in your life, the more you will have the feeling of fulfillment and accomplishment. Then you can truly rest inside yourself, satisfied that nothing is undone. You may still have unknown or hidden incompletions, but you relax because you have built the inner trust that when they reveal themselves, they will be completed.

The best thing you can do to enhance your self-trust is to develop the habit of taking responsibility for all your creations (which is everything in your life) and completing what you start. You are the one in charge and responsible for your life, and even if you've empowered something or someone else through blame or playing the victim, you are still in charge and responsible for your life. You can't get away from it.

Changing a habit takes time and patience. To build inner trust, relax and be gentle with yourself. And it's most important that you keep your word with yourself. Start by making one small agreement at a time and completing it. Do yourself a big favor and start now to develop the habit of completion. Completing what you put in motion is so important, as it is the destiny of each human being to complete. This is why the focus of the human consciousness is one of completion.

I cannot emphasize enough that completing what you start is one of the most worthwhile things you can do for your health and well-being. It's a joyful process because, as you complete, the unconscious starts clearing, your energy is returned to you, and you begin to live in the present, making conscious decisions and completing them on the spot. When the Bible says that the evil of today is enough (Matthew 6:34), it is telling us not to put things off until tomorrow.

No matter how beautiful something looks in the world, no matter how it glitters or how glamorous it is, it's always going to corrupt and decay. You're the one who is going to have to continue to maintain it, and that takes your energy. So make sure that it is important enough for you to put your energy into in a purposeful way, or drop it so you can go on to complete other things.

When you do choose to do something, do it with joy. Do it with a sense of completeness. It's preferable not to leave anything hanging out as incomplete because it will drop into the unconscious and be a drag on your energy later on. It is likely to give you a subtle sense of discomfort when you really should be comfortable doing anything, anytime, all the time, with anybody.

We don't like to think about our incompletions. So what we have not completed gets pushed down into an unconscious realm inside of us. Although that realm doesn't see, doesn't hear, and doesn't think or feel because it is asleep, it does have information and it does pull on our energy. You can feel when it's time to do something in an area you have been procrastinating about or avoiding. As you approach that area, you will start to get tired, achy, and sometimes you will even start nodding off because you are in the area that is sleeping.

Instead of going to sleep, that is exactly the time for you to stay present and awake, for you have arrived at the area in your consciousness where you have been avoiding living. You have found the area inside you that is unconscious, that's not aware, that's sleeping, and that has a large amount of your energy locked into it. Just imagine getting that energy loose and free!

*I cannot emphasize enough that completing what you start is one of the most worthwhile things you can do for your health and well-being.*

You can begin to free that energy in this moment, by moving your body into action and starting the process of completion. As you start to do this, you will feel the energy coming loose and free inside you, and you may find that all sorts of aches and pains will release. This is a healing action, not necessarily healing in terms of disease, but certainly healing in terms of completing your life patterns and goals. It's so extremely important because, as an area inside you that was asleep awakens, your energy stops leaking away into it and becomes immediately available to you as a conscious, awake person.

It's not doing that makes you tired. It is the going back and forth, and thinking, "Should I, or shouldn't I?" that wears you out. Only rarely does the physical body get honest-to-goodness tired, but it frequently gets exhausted from the mental and emotional struggle inside of us. As soon as you move on completing something, the energy is made available to you. The doing process is one of physically taking your body and moving and completing. You'll find you will have all the energy you need supplied to you when you work within the consciousness of completion.

Energy follows thought, and that energy will always go towards completion. So it's wise to keep moving towards completion; otherwise, our energy gets backed up and misdirected and will cause us to become tired, and sometimes quite ill. Because energy follows thought, my advice has always been to hold thoughts that uplift you. Hold images in your mind that you want more of. Be careful what you ask for because if you get it, you also get what goes with it. This is fine if, when it does come your way, you are prepared to handle it to completion.

The wonderful news is that the master key to completion is in our hands. We are the ones that decide when something is complete or finished, and we can declare it so. It's when we do not make the decision—when we do not choose to decide—that we can have problems with ourselves. You see, when we don't choose, a decision is still made for us—by default.

*Only rarely does the physical body get honest-to-goodness tired, but it frequently gets exhausted from the mental and emotional struggle inside of us. As soon as you move on completing something, the energy is made available to you.*

When you find that you don't have enough energy, when you're feeling tired and you don't know why, I would start to take a look at what you've started and haven't completed. We rarely sit down to eat a meal and think that we are not going to finish it or leave our home without an idea of our destination. We seem to always have a goal out there that we're striving to reach and bring to completion.

Goodness, we start so many projects! Those projects are not only started physically, but they can also be started in our minds and in our emotions. When we begin the project, it always seems like a good idea. Then, very often, another project that we "must do" comes to mind, and then another. The more projects you have going, the more thinly you spread yourself out.

Every project we put in motion demands a level of energy. We have no choice in the matter at all. The choice was already made when we said, "I'm going to do this project, and this one, and this one." Even though some projects are more important than others, as long as they are incomplete, they lie in the unconscious, equally. All of the "I'm going to do's" that are not finished are little hooks that hang out in our unconscious level wanting energy to feed them. The hooks then grab and pull on our energy level, and that's why we can feel so tired as if we are dragging ourselves through life.

How do you know these hooks are there when it is unconscious? You will know it indirectly. You may be having a conversation and something is mentioned in passing that you associate with something that is unfinished. This immediately triggers a release of energy—perhaps you become flushed or fidgety. You may even find yourself being judgmental, which then drains away even more of your energy.

*With each action of completeness, a tiny leak has been sealed. Keep going, joyfully, as with each small step of completion you will be reclaiming your energy.*

A way to prevent your energy from leaking into the unconscious is very simple and entirely in your hands—you intervene, consciously. For example, if you have an unread book sitting around for months and you know you are not going to get to it, pick it up, open it, and then close it and say, "I'm finished. I'm not going to read it anymore." That's all your consciousness has to hear—"I'm finished."

After all, don't we declare the end of things anyway? "This romance is over." "This marriage is through." "This job is finished." We are the ones who declare it. Don't you think it's marvelous that this is all our own ball game, in which we're the umpire, referee, batter, catcher, pitcher, and runner? However, it's important that you know that for this approach to work, you absolutely have to mean what you say.

As I said earlier on, energy follows thought. Even if the thought isn't complete, the energy keeps going and the energy doesn't care about your good intentions. So when you say you are finished with a half-read book that's been lying around for months, don't feel cheated that you didn't get out of it what you wanted. You weren't getting anything out of it while it was lying around anyway. It was draining you of your energy.

With each action of completeness, a tiny leak has been sealed. Keep going, joyfully, as with each small step of completion you will be reclaiming your energy.

# Principle 6

# Talking Yourself into Greater Vitality and Health

The concept of total wellness recognizes that our every thought, word, and behavior affects our greater health and well-being. And we, in turn, are affected not only emotionally but also physically and spiritually.

*Greg Anderson*

We condition ourselves by what we tell ourselves. Mostly, we tell ourselves what we don't really want or need to hear—how we are a failure, that we don't feel good or look good, that nothing is working, and that our life is going to hell. It's so funny because if we can tell ourselves the bad stuff, surely we can tell ourselves the good stuff. After all, we are the ones making up the stories, so why not tell ourselves the stories that will lift us and move us into greater health and loving?

You are in charge of what you say to yourself. You can say that your life is full of health, wealth, and happiness; abundance, prosperity, and riches; loving, caring, and sharing; and the joy of touching to others with that fullness. That story is, in actuality, closer to the truth of who you are and will manifest for you because as you think in your heart, you will become.

Why even be concerned about what somebody else is saying or thinking? It truly doesn't matter what I or anyone else says. What matters is what you say to yourself, and I fully support you saying good things to yourself and lifting and encouraging yourself.

One way we undermine ourselves and stay stuck in the past is through the "story" we tell ourselves about our lives. We seek an

*If you don't keep the agreement with yourself when you agree to do something, your body won't keep agreements with you when you tell it to do something. We're training it in disobedience continuously, and in disobedience we find illness.*

explanation for why we are the way we are in order to justify our behavior. However, for the most part, the story is fiction. There will be just enough truth to give it credibility, of course. But when we live our lives based on our made-up story, we are essentially living an illusion. In order to have an authentic life, we need to dismantle that illusion and leave behind our story of restriction and contraction, and we need to tell ourselves something new and uplifting.

*No matter what or whom you blame or feel a victim to, the responsibility always begins and ends with you.*

What is the story you tell yourself about why you are not as healthy as you'd like to be? Does the story start at birth? In childhood? In more recent years? Is it related to lack—not enough love, money, or attention? When in doubt, you can always blame your religion, your culture, or your beliefs to explain why you have closed down and contracted.

No matter what or whom you blame or feel a victim to, the responsibility always begins and ends with you. As you think about your story, be aware of the consistent theme that emerges. Usually, there is a point at which you began to feel like a victim. What judgments did you make—and perhaps are still making—about yourself, about others, about the world, about God?

As you think about it and take a good look, be scientific, not emotional, because you can mess around with yourself emotionally telling yourself how "no good" you are. Instead, sit down and say, "Okay, here's what I did," and start to write it down. "And here's the feelings I had with it, and here's what I thought with that." Make it all matter-of-fact. Now ask yourself what you can do to change that, either to your upliftment or to change it out of your life—transform it. Ask yourself some intelligent questions, because if you keep asking or telling yourself negative stuff, that's all you'll have to work with.

Break the cycle by inserting an intelligent response in with the emotional responses. That way you set up a positive emotional response ahead of the possibility of having something negative to say to yourself. It can be as simple as saying, "I forgive myself for holding onto grudges against so-and-so and I now let it go."

Many people see themselves as the sum of the past, the result of everything they've accumulated along the way. That's one way to look at life. I prefer to look at it another way. As I see it, the person I am today is perfectly positioned for my future. The future, not the past, has conspired to put me where I am in this moment, in this place, in this position in my life, so that I can claim the potential that awaits me.

You, too, are perfectly placed for your future. From that perspective, you can tell yourself the story of your success with your health. Take a piece of paper in a journal and start to write down the future story of your success in the area of your health, being as specific as you can. Don't hold back. See, hear, feel your new attitude and new approach as if you are already living it.

Be sure to make this a success story. Give it a happy ending. It is a quirk of human nature that even when the possibilities are endless, as they are in fantasy, we tend to imagine ourselves losing. While making up your story, be happy—no, be joyous—as you contemplate the best outcome for yourself.

With a little bit of altitude, perhaps you can understand that you have made up a story about your past. The key to note is that your story is made up. Certain things happened, of course, but you embellished them, borrowed some family and cultural traits, threw in a few expectations and judgments, added a pinch of hurt feelings, and then made up a philosophy to justify your decisions and actions. Now you can make up a new story, with a new philosophy, and begin to live it.

First, you need to stop criticizing yourself by saying things like, "Why did I do that? I shouldn't have done that!" because it sets up a cycle of negativity. It's a much better idea to say nice, positive things to yourself to balance the negative things you may have been saying to yourself for most of your life.

There is a very important thing that you can easily say to yourself. Whenever you do something that you feel isn't good, or you judge yourself, tell yourself, "Next time, I'll do better." Give yourself a break. Instead of beating yourself up, just say, "Next time, I'll do better." If we can program ourselves negatively by saying, "I'm no good," or "I'm bad," we can certainly program ourselves to say, "I'm good and I can do good things." That new programming will start to have you doing better the next time.

*The reason this principle of self-talking works so well is because of loving and the expression of loving.*

The reason this principle of self-talking works so well is because of loving and the expression of loving. If you find yourself feeling down or negative, just say to yourself, in your mind, "I'm happy. I'm happy." It's highly likely that in a short while your energy will start to move upwards. You were the one that made it happen by what you told yourself. Or if you find yourself in a situation you are emotionally caught up in, it could be with your family or at work, sometimes it's best just to say in your mind, "I release myself from their karma," and then let it go.

It's important that you watch what you say to yourself because the basic self accepts everything you say quite literally. If you say to yourself that you're "dying" for a cigarette, your basic self will accept it. At that point, the basic self erroneously equates quitting smoking with dying. It will feed back to you, "I'll die if I don't have a cigarette," until you reeducate it. So affirm life and speak kind words to yourself.

Part of the basic foundation of spiritual love is the expression of kindness. It is important to always speak kind words to one another and especially to yourself. It's important that you do let the greater love—not the love of man, but the love that comes from God—flow through you in your expression to yourself and others. It is this love that you must continually attempt to bring forward. Affirm your goodness because that is closer to the truth of who you are, and as you align inside with that truth, health and happiness will be the result.

# Principle 7

# We Live and Die
# at the Cell Level

The cell is immortal. As far as we know, the pulsation of life can go on forever.

*Dr. Alexis Carrell, Nobel Prize Winner*

Cells are the miracle of evolution. We come from just one single cell—the fertilized egg. Cells are very small, but for their size they are the most complex objects in the universe. Each of us is essentially a society of billions of cells that govern everything, from movement to memory and imagination. Cells can do a remarkable number of different things yet, in spite of the apparent difference between, for example, a nerve cell and a skin cell, they work by the same basic principles.

*Lewis Wolpert*

*Health is not so much about the food, or the nutrition in the food, it's more about how the cell level is energized, through clean blood and good oxygen—that's what brings life and vitality. When that's not happening, we get sluggish, lethargic, and we start dying. Literally, we start dying. We live and die at the cell level.*

Spirit enters into us first through the breath, then the nerves, blood, muscles, and then into the bones. The breath is a key to letting in the Spirit. If the blood becomes polluted, primarily through the acid-forming substances we introduce into the body, this acid will gather around the poles of the cells and corrode them, and the body will start to deteriorate and degenerate. As it starts to do that, you experience what we call dis-ease or disease.

If you get the idea of how cells degenerate really clear you'll start breathing more deeply, using your lungs more fully. You'll also be very careful about polluting your bloodstream, making it toxic through eating foods that are over-acidic. You'll start reaching for balance and harmony in your life.

It is known that a thought can alter structure and form in the body, and that negative thinking can poison the body systems very fast. We know that emotional disturbance, where negative emotions keep flooding the body with the hormones of disagreement, will make the body toxic. If the body is toxic, the cells stop vibrating harmoniously, and that affects the nerve responses.

*Cells don't die. They change their frequency and move to essence. The cell is a duplicate of the cosmos. That means you have full access to cosmic awareness within you, right now.*

There are no incurable diseases, only incurable people. Every seven to eleven years, we pretty much replace all the cells in the body. So, it really is up to us whether we're going to regenerate or degenerate.

Cells have a north pole and they have a south pole. The cells get their energy from the same place that a tree gets it—the sun and the essence of the air around us. If the air around us has life, and we can learn to utilize that efficiently, we can increase the ability of the blood to wash the cells and remove the corrosion off the ends of the poles of the cell, and the cell will keep regenerating itself, because it's a spiritual form. It's a divine form.

Cells don't die. They change their frequency and move to essence. The cell is a duplicate of the cosmos. That means you have full access to cosmic awareness within you, right now. Cells are fused with the energy of the material world; they find a corporal form and it grows into what we call our physical body. When the physical body dies, those cells remove themselves and go back to essence.

We could say that we are in optimum health when our cells are in love with one another, because in this loving they communicate clearly to maintain our physical body. Without this communication, they would disintegrate and we would disappear into another form of energy.

Another way to look at this is that we are in good health when our cells are at ease with each other, which is a perfect relationship. When those relationships go out of balance, we have anger, anxiety, repression, and other negative emotions. But even those negative emotions, if we use them correctly, can point the way back into perfect balance.

The cell has both a positive and negative vibration. When the cell has a positive vibration, there is health. When a negative starts to overtake or superimpose itself over the positive, there is illness. If we go along in life and we think about illness, over and over, like, "Oh, God! I'm going to have cancer," as we keep doing that, we are actually doing a form of meditation. What we meditate upon, we become and eventually, it manifests in the body.

The set up for the negative vibration to enter the body can also happen with the loss of a loved one or getting fired from work. A form of grief sets in and finds its way to the darkest part of the consciousness in the body and that will be located in a part of the cell. The more you focus upon your grief (not allowing the grieving which is the release, but, instead, focusing on the negative upset), the more the negative polarity of the cell takes over the positive and, right there, you have the fundamental basis for all illness in the body.

*If we can stimulate nerves and cells and get them vibrating at a higher rate, which can be done through using healing sounds, holding the images in our minds that we want more of, etc., then that positive vibration moves the cell back into balance.*

If we can stimulate nerves and cells and get them vibrating at a higher rate, which can be done through using healing sounds, holding the images in our minds that we want more of, etc., then that positive vibration moves the cell back into balance. Our challenge is to find balance in our body at all times, in every situation.

Another big key to health is that at the moment when you're contracting—for example, somebody hurt your feelings and you tighten your body—at that moment you have to cut the knot of contraction and expand. This is not to be done later on when you start feeling better, but immediately upon the moment of contraction. For example, when somebody cuts you off in traffic, or takes your parking place, or someone is rude or inconsiderate to you, rather than contracting, closing down, and getting upset, you might say to yourself, "Wait just a second! I'm not going to do that to myself because later I am going to get sick." Instead, you expand, relax, breathe, and move yourself into a loving vibration.

So often people have said to me, "But I have a right to be upset about that!" Yes, you do have a right to be upset. But it's not smart to exercise that right because there will be consequences to your health later on. The bad news is that a lot of these consequences do not appear immediately, and you're going to wonder when you set yourself up for that when they occur. It could be many years later that the consequences appear.

It's not like putting your hand on a hot stove, where it's immediate feedback, and you say, "Ouch! I won't be doing that again!" Yet, in these situations I am describing, it would be healthier for you to say just that, because the cells in the body react the way you react, and you can contract right into the bones. Contraction is the opposite of flow and openness, so it's to your benefit to continually watch where you place your focus.

*If we start listening to the wisdom of the body when pain in our bodies shows up, and we hold with it, images will start coming out of the cell levels.*

When negative emotions do arise, sacrifice them on the altar of love. Transmute the energy from anger to love. You can say, "I love this," whether you feel the love or not, because at the very least you are facing the right direction. That way, you won't have to clear the upsetting energy as it's now been transmuted to loving energy. So, as much upset as you had before, you have now got that much more love. I would suggest you make sure that all the cells of your body are feeling that loving, caring, and nurturing, because you're living in there, and you want your body to serve as the temple of your own countenance, your own Spirit, in the best way possible.

If we start listening to the wisdom of the body when pain in our bodies shows up, and we hold with it, images will start coming out of the cell levels. When they surface, don't say, "I'm still angry." Say instead, "Okay, God bless that one, you're gone." Then you have disciplined yourself to perceive and observe the world through loving. Then it doesn't matter what happens, because in a consciousness of loving, it's all going to be fine.

Keep in mind that everything can point you to God. Use every health situation to your advantage. Someone told me recently that they didn't understand clearly how they could use their asthma to their advantage. The how is something you have to come up with. I had asthma for 17 years. It took me 17 years to learn how to use it positively. I would run my entire family with my asthma attacks. I could bring the whole family to a stop. So, as I saw it, it was to my advantage to have asthma while I had it.

Had I known better I could have just asked for what I wanted but I needed to understand my emotional relationship with my family, first. My asthma was a crying out for love. When I saw how that worked, I never had to have asthma again. I wouldn't have had to create something that would hurt my lungs in order to get love.

Asthma can come from allergies to food. It's not necessarily karmic. The predisposition towards the asthma is karmic. I still have asthma, I just no longer experience it. It's in my system and I could produce it if I wanted to. I also know how not to produce it.

The foods that will irritate the lungs, the throat, and other parts of our body, will usually be the foods that we like the most—because we're addicted to foods that we like. When we eat the food, the allergy in the system stops. When the food is no longer effective in the body, the allergy kicks back up again—usually worse than before. When we eat that food again, the body quiets down.

That explains to you, in a very simple and general way, the addictions you may develop through allergies to food, alcohol, smoking, etc. Note that the majority of allergies go very many levels deep into the body. As one layer comes out, we feel it go away and we experience relief. Then something from a deeper cell level memory comes up and the allergy is kicked off again. If this applies to you, go deeper with it. Eventually the healing will take place.

On a path towards healing, I suggest starting with the allergies and getting those out of the way. Nutrition is a big part of this. Not just any kind of nutrition, but the correct kind for you. It may not be the same for anybody else. And it will change as you go through the stages of a healing process.

Cell level memory will start surfacing in these healing processes. You may have gotten over the symptoms, but you didn't get the healing. The healings have to come within a certain time of the disease before it goes into pathology and causes a cell change. I haven't found anything that can't be reversed. But the things that will reverse it need to be done, and for the most part it is not easy or pleasant. Often, you have to change your environment, change what you eat, change your friends, and change the way you go about healing yourself.

The bottom line of our existence is that we want to feel good, and the only thing that is good is God. What we really want is to feel God. The way we feel God is through loving. God is love. So it all boils down to a crying out for love—for that good feeling and connection with God.

We may be able to find that connection with other people, but that's not the everlasting God, and it may end in death or divorce. Whereas the connection with God goes into eternal life, so it's quite obvious to me where I would choose to place my attention.

God is both quality and quantity. Down here on the planet, it is always more of one than the other, but you won't get both, fully, at one time, because that would make it complete here and we wouldn't die. We're dying, so it's not complete. So we go towards the completeness of the one Spirit of God. Once we find that as an idea or a feeling, disease leaves the body.

When the energy of Spirit starts to come present, it comes in through the air, in through us and into the Soul. It's an invisible energy from God, and it starts to permeate the cell levels, which in turn starts to purify and clean us out. But you've got to receive it. You've got to be open and allow it to happen. And you've got to take whatever healing is available to you.

You may ask, "How do I take it?" You take it by removing the blocks in your consciousness to life, by allowing them to surface, taking responsibility for them, and loving them and forgiving yourself for judging them.

When you go right down to the cell level, you'll find that it has fire in it. We know that it has light, but what produces the light is a fire. These elements of light and fire living in us hold our cell-level memory. That's how we form our habits. Your perpetuating and continually repeating the same thing maintains those habits. Once you understand that, it is very easy to give these elements of light and fire different food. You can begin to change their behavior by changing your diet. And then changing your mental, emotional, and physical behavior is also "food" for your cells and influences the energy flow into the cell and it starts to change. Positive behavior will produce positive results.

Spiritual exercises and meditation will not necessarily transmute cell-level conditions as much as conscious awareness does by our thinking and acting upon the positive attributes of our life. We essentially feed the cell with the vibrations of regeneration, vitality, and life through the way we live. But that doesn't necessarily rejuvenate us—we also have to go through a change in consciousness before the new pattern of vitality holds.

Introducing stem cells into the body is an attempt to affect that sort of change. However, the body's systems are currently rejecting them faster than the new vibration can transmute into the cell structure. My approach and suggestion to all of this is to keep altering our consciousness into the divine and increase our vibratory rate that way. If we want to break the routines and habits that are no longer working for us, we have to do things in a radical way from time to time, in order to break up the distribution of energy within the cell. For example, we don't want a lot of cells functionally devoted towards addictive behavior. We want our cells devoted to creatively visualizing and making life better. We want just a very small amount of ourselves devoted to habitual routines—ones that work for us, of course.

We need to learn to refocus back on the Godness within us, which is the goodness. I say it in this way; "I'm keeping my eyes on you, Lord, only you." You may ask, what about the pain? "I'm keeping my eyes on you Lord, only you." That's my answer to the pain,

*The bottom line of our existence is that we want to feel good, and the only thing that is good is God. What we really want is to feel God. The way we feel God is through loving.*

because, if you look at the Lord, there is freedom. Then you learn to let that freedom move through the cells of the body. As the freedom moves through the cells of the body they catch the fire of the Spirit. As I've mentioned, at the root of each cell, there's fire or flame. It's not the fire you get when you light a match; it's a spiritual fire.

When you open the cell, fire connects with the divine Spirit flowing into you, the whole body will usually have a rush of heat. Then you relax and receive. Your body and cells are being transformed into a higher vibration and new patterns of behavior. You relax—let go, and be patient—let God. Why? You never know when God's going to do it. So far, He's never been on my schedule. But He's always been on schedule. When I move to that, the healing just happens. I've found out that if I want an easy life, I just stay in the flow of being relaxed and patient.

*Give from the spiritual heart, and you'll be amazed at how Spirit takes care of its own. It will bring in the right food; it will absorb it and assimilate it for your greatest health.*

Give from the spiritual heart, and you'll be amazed at how Spirit takes care of its own. It will bring in the right food; it will absorb it and assimilate it for your greatest health. Once you recognize the God-quality within, you move through life in a neutral state. In the neutral state, you then are master of all things around you, and all you have to do is stay within the boundaries of neutrality, neither saying "yes" here, "no" there, or "good" or "bad," or "happiness" or "depression," but just seeing "what is" as it comes your way.

The attitude that we place on top of our desires is what we need to check, to make sure it is healthy for us. If you say, "I desire good health; I desire good health," what kind of resistance are you placing? You're fortifying bad health. You're better off to say, "All things come my way in a right and proper direction. I am that I am. Here I am, God."

# Principle 8

# There is Only One Energy and That Energy is Love

**The power of love to change bodies is legendary, built into folklore, common sense, and everyday experience. Love moves the flesh, it pushes matter around. Throughout history, "tender loving care" has uniformly been recognized as a valuable element in healing.**

*Larry Dossey, M.D.*

*A lot of people want to talk about how the energy is good or bad. What they ought to do is look inside of themselves and see how the energy is inside of them, because the energy inside is the energy out there, available equally to all of us.*

People often say that love will cure the world. But this is not exactly true. It is loving that cures the world. Loving is action. Loving is manifestation. Loving is movement. Loving is the consciousness of giving.

It is important to keep moving and not let yourself get stuck and stagnant in any aspect of your life. Keep moving in the direction of your loving. Love is difficult to define. We might say that love is the essence that brings forces together and holds them in a "position" relative to one another. When we look at things simply, we can say that our cells are "in love" with one another, because they stand together. If they weren't, they would separate from one another.

The experience of love cannot come from a book or be contained in words. It can only be experienced. Many people use the words of the Bible or other sacred texts as a weapon against others, and they destroy just as effectively as if they were using knives or swords or guns. In loving, no one has to defend anything or attack anything. No one has to win; no one has to lose. In loving, if you lose, the winner will help you pick up the pieces.

Love is given to everyone, just as the sun shines on everyone. Not everyone, however, wants to stand in the sun. You are the one who determines the level of your experience with love. Love sits by you until that time when you will let love flow through. Letting love flow through is very easy. All you do is move to a neutral position—not one of belief or disbelief, not one of judgment or prejudice, but one of receptivity. As soon as you judge, you strike against love.

Take the attitude that no matter where you look, no matter what you see, it is a manifestation of love. That which you see is love in front of you. Love may be many different sizes, shapes, and forms, but it is all love. If you enter your inner world in love, and you maintain that love, you can live more freely and effortlessly.

When you do not love, you do not fully live. If you do not fully live, God cannot pour the fullness of His energies through you into the world. Those of you who know of the love within and are so filled with it, can give of this love so that others may awaken to it. In this way, humankind might become more tender and loving.

You do not have to love personalities. People are not their personalities. You are not your personality. You know that you are not your mind; it changes too often. Your emotions go up and down. Your body gets old too fast and develops all sorts of aches and pains. Then what are you? You are living love. You always have been. Let your loving lead you into awakening and the discovery of what you already are.

When love comes to you, don't refuse it by thinking you are not worthy. You are worthy, or love couldn't come your way. There is a "taker" part in everyone that says, "But when do I get mine?" That's the ego speaking. Give love. Give silently. Don't tell people what to do. Instead, just support them with your love. That's the best gift of all.

The purest love is always unconditional. There are no strings, no conditions, and no expectations of any return. The giving is pure. If you give 100 percent and love totally, you need no return. If you love 100 percent, you can bring healing to anything.

When you come from the heart, from the center of love, you do not come from the mind or emotions. You do not come from the ego, attempting to control others or force anything down their throats. If you want pure love, then go to where pure love resides. Pure love is the Soul. It is inside you and needs no interpretation.

Now is the only moment. This is it. This is all there is. Enjoy it. You can still have aspirations and plans and visions; just place them where you can realistically handle them, and that starts with right here and now. Loving is a matter of giving yourself 100 percent at any moment. If you are married, give 100 percent to the marriage and to your spouse.

If you hold back or place conditions on the marriage, and keep part of your loving in reserve, you will never know what that marriage could have been. You will never know where the expression of loving could have led you. If you love 99 percent and do not go the full 100 percent, you will end up in lack. There will be something lacking and you will know it. When you investigate and explore loving 100 percent, there is no unknown area and thus no fear.

The next time you are in front of a mirror, look at yourself. Look yourself in the eye. If you don't like what you see, it's just another aspect of yourself for you to love. If you start to feel the quality of loving drop away or go stagnant, it's time to stop and take another close look at what you are doing. Perhaps you forgot to love where you are. Truly, truly, truly, you must love everything you see.

*Love is given to everyone, just as the sun shines on everyone. Not everyone, however, wants to stand in the sun. You are the one who determines the level of your experience with love. Love sits by you until that time when you will let love flow through.*

There is never a good enough reason to take away your loving. You have the ability not to care for people's personalities and still love every human being for who they are. You can prefer not to be involved with someone acting negatively and still love the person even if the action is not to your liking. Keep in mind that this world is conditioned energy, and what you are reaching for is a loving that is unconditional. That loving is always available, but you must be available to it, without conditions.

Love yourself for being "hardheaded." Love yourself for not being able to play a guitar and sing and write music. Love yourself for being a "good-for-nothing." You are such a lovely one. Love yourself, even when you don't know what's going on. Even when you don't feel like loving, love the feeling of not feeling loving. There is no way you can separate yourself from love and maintain freedom. The only way to true freedom is to love it all.

You can be everything you want to be as soon as you unconditionally become unconditional. Loving is the key: total, unconditional loving. If you can't love somebody, it's best to say, "I don't know who they are." That's a clear, precise, and honest statement, because if you don't love someone, you really don't know who they are. The person you criticize, the one you put down, is not known to you. Anyone who is truly known to you is loved.

*Now is the only moment. This is it. This is all there is. Enjoy it. You can still have aspirations and plans and visions; just place them where you can realistically handle them, and that starts with right here and now.*

Don't lose in your fantasy. Always win in your fantasy because you're making it up. Don't make it up bad, make it up good. Although you may not know it yet, God's plan for you, for your neighbor, and for the world is perfect. When you choose to accept rather than demand change, when you chose to support rather than criticize, when you choose to love rather than hurt, that is when something inside you stands up and cheers.

Have you ever found that the only good thing about suffering is when it stops? When the suffering stops, you feel that you have learned something, so you think that the suffering was good for you. But you could have learned without the suffering.

How do you let go of those things in your consciousness that no longer serve you? The answer is to open up to greater love. Love will go in and stir the pain that you've locked away from even yourself. As it is stirred, it will begin to surface and release. You have the ability to raise yourself. Don't contract from your experiences. Bless them. Love them. They are your ladders into expansion and higher consciousness.

You do not have to force your awakening or push the speed of your unfoldment. You can, however, assist the process by loving yourself every step of the way, and by treating the people around you with kindness and honesty. There's nothing for you to do but be natural, and the most natural, God-like act is simply loving.

When you confront your challenges in life, rise to the highest point within you, which is love. There, you will find the key to the

Kingdom. But there is a catch. The love must encompass all things. You must love your depression, love your despair, love your anger, love your confusion, and love your upset.

If you bring irritation to people, love the irritation and the people. Sometimes you are a master of irritation. Wouldn't you rather be a master of love? When you awaken each morning, it might be nice if you asked for the peace of God to be with you and all that you touch that day. If you ask for attunement each day, it will change the quality of your life. If you are one with God's consciousness, no person can come against you. To find the peace within, it is often necessary to become quiet, so that you can hear the voice of love from within.

Don't resist the negativity within you. Love it. Loving will purify and lift all negativity.

If you have a negative thought, love the idea of having a negative thought. That is the way to turn a stumbling block into a stepping-stone. Or you can say, "I don't have to travel that path," and then you don't. Instead, you can let love lead you in another direction.

You have the right to choose your direction. In fact, once you let love lead, it is your duty. If you don't perform this duty, then the consequences lead you. Consequences are your reaction instead of your action. Love your consequences. They are your opportunity to learn. They are your opportunity to gain wisdom. They are your opportunity to properly identify with what is true.

When you close yourself off, you can become depressed because you miss the loving you once experienced. If you cannot get in touch with and share the loving that is present for you, then share your depression and anxiety. Treat your loving and your depression as equal. Anxiety, love, depression, and happiness must all be treated equally. When you do, there can be no place for anything "better" or "worse" inside you, so judgment ceases to have power in your consciousness. When you treat your depression the same as your loving, then neither has more power than the other does, and you are free to choose the expression you want.

You're going to be another day older whether you do anything today or not. So this day, why not say, "I love you whether or not you love me." That's the beginning of self-mastery. You'll have the freedom inside you to say, "I love you when you're here. I love you when you're not here. If I never see you again, I'll still love you. If you go, I'll miss you, but that's the part of me that's conditioned to miss. I'll get over it because I'm going to go on loving." Sometimes you feel like you can't go on, but you do. Look at all the times you've said, "I'll never live through this," and here you are, living through it.

*You can be everything you want to be as soon as you unconditionally become unconditional. Loving is the key: total, unconditional loving.*

When someone is angry or is fighting with you, often the easiest demonstration of your love is to be silent. That's one way to win, but it only works if you truly maintain your center of love. You give that love in a pure way, continuously, like the pulling of a golden silk thread. It's the best way to win, because the other person gets to win too.

Maintain your loving just a little while longer than you think you need to. Then you are becoming master of yourself. When you try to master someone else, you haven't mastered yourself. You become a taker. Then you are out of your center of love, for loving is a giving action. When you have mastered yourself, you do not have to go any further. You don't have to master anybody else to prove you've mastered yourself.

Living love is loving yourself first, so that you can love others. It's taking care of yourself, so that you can help take care of others. It's doing those things that are good for you, so that you'll be happy, healthy, and a joy to be with. Love is everywhere when there is loving in you.

To be healthy physically, be healthy in your emotions, your actions, your mind, your thoughts, your heart. Speak kind words to yourself and to others. Do those things that will support your body physically. Reach out and touch others. Take responsibility for your actions, and handle your responsibilities in an appropriate manner.

There is nothing wrong with being selfish. Eating and getting proper rest are selfish for the body, thinking nice thoughts is selfish for the mind, feeling good is selfish for the emotions, and doing spiritual exercises to rouse the Soul that may be sleeping is selfish for the Spirit. Those are all healthy activities. If other people fit in with your plan for taking care of yourself, that can be fantastic. If they undermine the plan, let them go their own way. Let them go in love, with good thoughts and good feelings towards them—but let them go if they do not support you in those things that are good for you. Experience the devotion to yourself that allows you to take care of yourself.

Going to a doctor is a form of love. It's a way of saying that you are starting to take better care of yourself, and taking care of yourself is loving yourself. This physical body is truly a temple of the Spirit. And you can build your body so that it does not become a heavy body, but a light body, so that the Spirit can work more closely with you.

When you reach a harmony within yourself, you can take cells that have been out of balance and, by placing a ring of love around them, hold them in balance for five or ten years. Love and joy and happiness can change the frequency of cell structure from the "doom and gloom" of a cell disintegrating to a lilting, joyful quality of a cell lifting into balance and harmony.

Take care of yourself on all levels. Do those things that will be uplifting. Be with other people who are following the upward path. Be loving to yourself and to others. A key to breaking free is to love yourself and to love each experience that comes to you whether it appears to be negative or positive. Love it all equally. Love it all, own it all—and you will be free.

Enough love will handle all things. If you are having difficulty handling something, you don't have enough love for that thing. So your next step is laid out right in front of you: get some more love. If there are still areas of your life that cause you difficulty, bless them. Indeed, those areas are your blessings because they move you to seek the Kingdom of God. If all things were perfect here, you might forget all about your spiritual direction.

When you can look at your life in perspective, you will see the humor of it. Enjoy it. Enjoy yourself in all your escapades. When you do, it's easy for the loving to come present and manifest itself in everything you do. Love is the key—total, unconditional love. Even when you don't feel like loving, you love the feeling of not feeling like loving.

*Enough love will handle all things. If you are having difficulty handling something, you don't have enough love for that thing.*

When things are going badly, sit down and say, "I love me anyway." Even your negative experiences are gifts from Spirit to build your strength, your awareness, your empathy, and your loving. Thank God for them. When you are secure in your knowledge of God's love for you, you know that everything that happens is to lift you and move you closer to your own divinity. I found out a long time ago that what the Lord does is perfect, and there is nothing designed to hurt or harm you.

Love your karma also. It is your opportunity to learn and to gain wisdom. By loving even your negative creations, you can shift their energy and release karma. You have the opportunity to change the karmic flow of your life through your ability to be loving. By loving the God in yourself and others, you can move into a path of greater unfoldment. Instead of looking at the factors of your life and saying, "That's my karma, so I can't help it," you might say, "That's my karma, and I will fulfill it so I am free." Through loving, you can complete your karma.

There is only one energy. My concept of energy is a word called "love." And we could add, "unconditional." The most profound thing I have found out about this unconditional love is that it is no more present in one person than it is in another, and it allows each person to do with it what they will. Now it's remarkable that you have a substance that is life-giving, life-sustaining, and is life, and it will let you corrupt it and let you do anything with it you want to—even come back in line with it.

Since this one energy is always a source, and always (all ways) a supply, there's only one thing left to do with this whole process called life, and that's just have a good laugh about it! It's hilarious to think that we have within us the absolute essence of perfection, and we're messing around with it. We're getting sick, having problems, having despair, and worrying about things going on in life, and it's all under a direction of something that's going to handle it all anyway.

Take good care of yourself; that's another way to love yourself. Eat good foods. Exercise. Do those activities that keep you healthy. Put your physical choices and activities in a higher perspective so you see them as opportunities to love yourself more fully. If you want the spiritual flow to work unconditionally, then you must let it flow unconditionally. No modifications. No conditions. No deals. Just keep it open. If you move from a state of tension, you will be blocked. If you always move from your center of relaxation, you will be free.

*When things are going badly, sit down and say, "I love me anyway." Even your negative experiences are gifts from Spirit to build your strength, your awareness, your empathy, and your loving.*

When you are loving unconditionally, you won't care what I do or what anyone else does. It's not that you care less, it's just that, in your own inner space, where everyone lives inside you, it is a healthy, wealthy, and happy place. I found out a long time ago that if I am out of harmony with anyone inside of me, then I am out of harmony with myself also. If you are carrying anyone inside you that you are judging, your thoughts and feelings about them are robbing you of your energy. Bring them into harmony through love and forgiveness, or keep them outside of your inner environment. I want my inner environment to be sacred, soft, and unconditionally loving so that I can return there often for nurturing and regeneration.

No one can create love. Love is. When it shows up, we drop everything and go with it because it never leads us astray. Love doesn't abuse or take advantage of others; love leads to God. Love is the bliss consciousness in the heart. It brings health and vitality. It brings the opportunity to have all things. Loving begins within each one of us, and health is loving who you really are. Since you already sit in the center of all things, why have anything else?

# Applying the Principles

As you read the eight spiritual principles of health and well-being, which one resonated most for you? Perhaps they all resonated, but to keep things simple and practical for yourself, consider choosing one of the principles, for a period of time, to focus on and apply to the way you live your life.

What follows in this section called *Applying the Principles* are three of the most common health situations and challenges we all face in today's culture. Read through them once to get an idea of the material. Then I suggest you read through them for a second time with a view to seeing how can you use the principle you have chosen to navigate through these three areas in order to create a healthier lifestyle for yourself.

For example, you may find that through applying the principle of completion (#5) in your life, you will considerably reduce your level of stress. Or by applying the principle of loving (#8), you may find a dramatic reduction in your need for sugar. Have fun and experiment with this.

As you read through the next section, it may be helpful for you to be aware of inflammation. Information about inflammation has come a long way since the ancient Latin description of Rubor, Calor, tumor, and dolor (redness, heat, swelling, and pain). We still have these symptoms with infection, but the much more significant issue is the internal, silent (below the perception of pain) inflammation, which is now looked upon as possibly the main factor precipitating chronic disease and aging.

Inflammation is a process in which our immune system releases compounds designed to heal trauma (for example, sunburn) and infection or to handle foreign substances, such as toxins from the environment. This is a healthy and normal response; however, when inflammation is chronic, it can severely weaken the tissues of the body.

An under-appreciated contributor to the whole body, silent inflammation is the balance of the intestinal tract. As 80% of our immune tissue lines the gut, an inflammatory diet activates the immune system as it passes through the digestive phases.

Pro-inflammatory foods include high fructose corn syrup, Advanced Glycation End Products (or AGEs, explained in section called "Less Sugar"), unhealthy animal fat or trans fats, high-carbohydrate refined sugar foods, and deep fried foods. Some natural anti-inflammatory nutrients are the Omega-3 fatty acids, phytochemicals, and antioxidants in berries, green tea, and quercitin (found in apples).

This is something you may want to check out with your healthcare professional. The most common measurement of silent inflammation is C-reactive protein or CRP.

As you read the following chapters realize that they are an overview and a vast oversimplification of what are complex biological processes. Perhaps in reading it you find a window into your own health situation or you find that one small step that takes you towards better health and well-being. Once again, we recommend that you consult with your healthcare professional before making any changes in your personal life as it pertains to your health. If you are seeking a deeper look at the subject matter covered in this section then consult the bibliography at the back of this book.

# Less Stress

Slow down and everything you are chasing will come around and catch you.

*John De Paola*

Sometimes the most important thing in a whole day is the rest we take between two deep breaths.

*Etty Hillesum*

Stress is an ignorant state. It believes that everything is an emergency. Nothing is that important.

*Natalie Goldberg*

Not all stress is bad. Stress can be to our advantage and work for us when we use it to grow stronger and more adaptable. This chapter is about the unnecessary stress that causes degeneration in the body. If you were to take just one small step towards greater health and well-being that could be maintained for the rest of your life, finding a way to reduce unnecessary self-induced stress would be a good one to take.

It used to be thought that our health was determined 80 percent by our genetics and 20 percent by our environment and lifestyle choices. Current thinking and research has reversed those percentages, and it is now widely thought that our health is determined 80 percent by our environment and lifestyle and 20 percent by our genetics. (More advanced thinking suggests that it's possible for us to change our genetic expression through our nutrient intake.)

What this tells us is that none of us need to be victims—there is a lot of power in our hands through the choices we make. One of those choices is not to flood our body with the hormones of disagreement. In other words, we can keep our emotional and mental stress to a minimum by not reacting negatively to outer events.

*Watch that you don't flood your emotional body with hormones from the glandular system.*

*We know that emotional disturbance, where you keep emotionally flooding your body with the hormones of disagreement, will make the body toxic.*

A few years ago, a Mayo Clinic heart study found that psychological stress was the strongest predictor of heart problems including cardiac arrests and heart attacks. Anxiety, chronic stress, and high blood pressure all raise the risk of cardiovascular disease. In addition, research shows that people who sleep only 6 hours a night have a 66 percent greater tendency towards hypertension.

In this chapter, let's take a brief look at the basics of the stress response that are most relevant to the material we are covering in this book. If you want to explore this more deeply, there are many sources of information on this subject, some of which are listed in the appendix.

In the early days of man, there was clean air, organic food, and fresh water, and humans had to walk and run everywhere they went. (As one prehistoric man commented to another in a New Yorker cartoon, "How come we're only living to 35 years old?") In addition to this abundance of natural food, there was also an abundance of natural predators—wild animals. Thus we developed the stress response as a survival mechanism to get out of danger as quickly as possible by moving—fast. That response is still in our genetics to this day. When our lives are in danger (for example, a fire in a building we are in), the body's response is to produce the hormones that get us to act quickly, either to put the fire out or to run. This response has been popularly called "fight or flight." When the danger passes and we get back to our cave, or house, safely, we relax (at least we are supposed to). The stress response has done its job.

The situation today is that, although fires and being chased by dangerous animals are rare, we still manage to turn the stress response on regularly—often several times a day—in response to traffic jams, someone cutting in front of us as we drive, an irritating co-worker, waiting a long time in line, our computer acting slowly, and our latte not having enough foam.

When we are stuck in traffic and we are getting upset because we are late for an appointment, our stress hormones are set in motion and say to us, "Move! Get going out of here." But we can't move. We are stuck in traffic, our seat belts are holding us in our car seats, and our hormones are circulating through our body wondering why we aren't moving. We are over stimulating our system. Over time, this causes a lot of wear and tear on the body.

The body doesn't discriminate between psychological stress—when we are worried about the economy, worried about our job, worried about everything—and physical stress—when we need to get out of the way of danger. If you are at work and someone is upsetting you, plus you dislike your job, the psychological stress of your upset is affecting you several times a day, if not all the time. Eventually, the cumulative effect on the body is enormous.

*We can keep our emotional and mental stress to a minimum by not reacting negatively to outer events.*

Keep in mind that the body is an extremely complex, sophisticated, and efficient communication system, a massive network which, when properly functioning, has every part communicating with every other part through its various systems. One of the key messengers in this communication system is called hormones.

When danger is perceived, real or imagined (real in the case of a fire or imagined where you see a snake in the grass that turns out to be a garden hose), the hypothalamus starts the stress response by communicating to the pituitary gland, a pea-sized gland attached to the base of the brain, through a hormone called CRF. The pituitary then releases a hormone called ACTH to the adrenal glands, which sit on top of the kidneys. The adrenals are capable of releasing several kinds of hormones, the most familiar of which is called adrenalin (epinephrine). Glucocorticoids are another hormone the adrenals secrete the most commonly known of which is called cortisol.

While the above is going on, there is a "hard-wired" signal from the hypothalamus, through the sympathetic nervous system, to the adrenal gland stimulating it to release adrenaline immediately. Thus, there are two responses to the stressor happening in the body simultaneously. The immediate shot of adrenaline through the nervous system (for example, reacting to a loud noise) and a slower response through the circulatory system involving cortisol when the stressor is more prolonged (for example a bad marriage).

When the stress response is triggered, because of a saber-toothed tiger, an angry spouse, a bothersome co-worker, or a negative fantasy, adrenalin is released. One of adrenalin's first jobs is to call for the production of glucose to give us a sugar boost so we have the energy we need to get moving. (Later, cortisol does this by a process called glucogenesis where it tells the liver to produce glucose from its stored amino acids.)

*The body doesn't discriminate between psychological stress—when we are worried about the economy, worried about our job, worried about everything—and physical stress—when we need to get out of the way of danger.*

The glucose is delivered through our circulatory system. The adrenaline goes to the heart and starts it pumping fast, constricting the arteries so the blood travels faster and with more force in order to deliver oxygen and energy to the brain, heart, and muscle cells. That's why during a stress response, we often find ourselves shaking, our heart beating faster, and breathing more rapidly. In this increase in cardiovascular (heart and blood vessels) output, the blood pressure goes up. Although blood is delivered with greater speed to the muscles, there is a decreased blood flow to the momentarily unessential parts of the body (digestive tract, kidneys, and skin).

A continued stress response keeps the cardiovascular system in this heightened state, wearing out the heart and arteries. What begins as a response to assist us, with prolonged use, becomes a detriment. If we perceive that the stressor is still present, we continue to activate the stress response. Adrenalin tends to fade within a few minutes or, at the longest, by the time we go to sleep. Cortisol, however, can stay elevated for hours, days, weeks, and longer, inducing the debilitating symptoms of chronic stress and adrenal depletion.

This is where our five keys for health fit in. They all work well as an antidote to the stress response.

### 1. Move your body—stretch, take a walk.

*This is one of the best ways to move the stress hormones through and out of the body.*

2. *Drink more water, good water, to keep the system flushed.*
   *Water cleanses the system and helps remove the toxicity from the*
   *stress hormones.*

3. *Watch that you don't flood your emotional body with*
   *hormones from the glandular system.*
   *The glandular system being referred to is the endocrine system and*
   *the interaction between the hypothalamus, pituitary, and adrenal*
   *glands commonly called the HPA axis.*

4. *Watch your thinking and create a system of self-talking that*
   *talks you into greater vitality and health.*
   *We can create stress just by thinking of potentially negative things.*
   *We can help mitigate this process by talking ourselves through the*
   *imagined situation to the other, positive side of it.*

5. *Keep the images in your mind that you want more of.*
   *This is vital to health and well-being and is covered in depth in*
   *Principle #2.*

Cortisol is particularly worthy of our attention because it is a
hormone that it is in touch with all the systems of the body.
Its appearance in the body is part of our normal day-to-day
functioning, but once activated in the system in response to stress,
its first job is to ensure the survival of the body, and it starts to shut
down every function that is not necessary for immediate survival.
For example, it tells the body to stop repairing tissue, because that
can be done later when the "danger" is past. It also tells the body to
forget about sex as that can be done later, too; otherwise, no sex—
forever. Perhaps you can now see why stress compromises the
repair and healing mechanisms of the body and is also associated
with low libido.

Cortisol also begins to shut down the immune system, ironically, for the same reason—survival. Fundamentally, the immune system consists of leukocytes and monocytes. These are white blood cells that spring to action and start killing off foreign invaders—unfriendly bacteria and viruses that attack the body. Cortisol puts the immune system on hold, and it even interferes with the communication system between the white cells. It can even go as far as to start killing the white cells. Cortisol takes its job very seriously.

Just take a moment to think of the effects of cortisol springing to action several times a day and unleashing the above effects, not necessarily over what is actually going on in our lives, but because of what we are thinking or imagining is going on—"Will I get fired?" "Will I have enough money?" "Are my children safe?" etc.

We can immediately see the benefits of holding thoughts in our mind we want more of and talking positively to ourselves. Our lifestyle choices, and how we use our minds, imagination, and emotions in our day-to-day life, can have a big influence on our health and well-being. Where does our unconscious come in on all of this? The unconscious can be looked at as a dumping ground for incomplete thoughts and emotions. *(To clear the unconscious see the chapter on free-form writing, page 243)*

Cortisol is also activated when we have inflammation in our bodies. Cortisol is a steroid. You can find it in creams to handle inflammation of the skin, and in certain cases of severe inflammation, it is injected into the body. In high doses it has the side effects we have mentioned above—compromised repair of tissue, shutting down of the immune system, promotion of diabetes, etc.

A typical, healthy, cortisol cycle in the body has a high point at around 8 am—it wakes us up. Then cortisol levels gradually decline throughout the day, until by evening with low cortisol in your body, you are ready to go to sleep. However, our propensity to find stress everywhere in our current lifestyle plays havoc with this natural cortisol cycle, commonly known as our circadian rhythm.

Those people who are unable to sleep regularly or who work a night shift tend to be the most severely affected by the disruption in this natural cycle.

A person under continual stress will invariably go to bed in the evening very tired, or exhausted, and instead of waking up by 8 a.m. may find themselves wide awake and alert at 2 a.m. This can happen because of taking caffeine in the late afternoon or evening or going to bed upset with someone. When the natural cortisol cycle is out of balance, the result is often tiredness and fatigue, because the body is not being allowed to rest.

*A continued stress response keeps the cardiovascular system in this heightened state, wearing out the heart and arteries. What begins as a response to assist us, with prolonged use, becomes a detriment.*

As part of the stress response, the adrenal glands also secrete hormones called mineralocorticoids that are involved in regulating the correct potassium and sodium levels for the body, which is also part of maintaining the body's electrolyte balance. Depleted adrenal glands can compromise this response and thus salt cravings can also be a part of being over-stressed.

Cortisol also restricts insulin. This is a reason why under chronic stress we start to have more sugar in the system that can eventually cause us to put on weight and, when left unchecked, can go into obesity and diabetes. Then there is chronic fatigue syndrome, and all sorts of other syndromes and conditions; the list goes on and on. Elevated cortisol can alter blood sugar levels, increase triglyceride and cholesterol levels, deplete minerals in our bones setting us up for osteoporosis, impair the immune system, reduce muscle mass, inhibit tissue regeneration, increase fat, impair memory, and destroy brain cells.

When you have too much cortisol in your system you have a shut-down immune system, and when you have too little cortisol, you have little or no energy. The body is constantly striving for homeostasis—a balanced state in which good health can flourish. Cells die when they move out of their homeostatic balance. As you've read before, we live and die at the cell level.

The HPA (hypothalamus, pituitary, adrenal) axis, mentioned above, is a system that's regulated by negative feedback loop. It's just like your heating system at home—once the target temperature is reached, it shuts off, and when it gets low, it kicks on. In a normally functioning body, when the stress event is over, the cortisol levels drop and the systems that had been turned off are turned back on. But when the system is out of balance, the systems that repair tissue and allow the body to fully function stay turned off.

*You are supposed to move, and that is why an effective way to deal with stress and upset is to move the body—walk, jog, run, or do push-ups—in order to move the energy through.*

What can we do about all of this? What changes to our lifestyle can we make to deal with stress? A number of years ago, there was a seminal article in The New York Times about stress. In it one of the top stress researchers in the country, Dr. Bruce McEwen, said that one of the most effective antidotes to stress is belly breathing.

Belly breathing is also called diaphragmatic breathing, and it involves relaxing and allowing the belly to expand with each inhalation. To start out, you can practice by lying down and putting your hand over your belly as you breathe. You can also put your hand on your chest to contrast breathing from your belly, which triggers a parasympathetic nervous system (relaxation) response, and breathing from your chest, which triggers a sympathetic nervous system (fight or flight) response.

The sympathetic and parasympathetic nervous systems are part of the autonomic nervous system. The autonomic nervous system controls the automatic functions of the body. Our heart beats automatically and most of our breathing is done without our conscious involvement. This is the autonomic system at work.

When under stress the sympathetic nervous system is geared to action, cortisol is released. As we've discussed, your heartbeat goes faster, your breathing becomes rapid, and you are ready to go. You are supposed to move, and that is why an effective way to deal with stress and upset is to move the body—walk, jog, run, or do push-ups—in order to move the energy through. Inactivity leads to adrenalin building up in the system, and it makes the body acidic. Deep breathing is also a good antidote to stress because it not only calms the body down but also alkalizes the body.

One easy thing you can do for your health is to maintain an active fitness program. The main dividing line between those who do well over the age of fifty, and those who don't, is whether or not you stay physically fit. Your fitness program doesn't have to be a competitive one, just one where your heart rate can be healthily increased and the muscles exercised. Something as simple as walking will do. The bloodstream is either the cesspool or the life giver. If it's a cesspool, you're dying in your own garbage. If it's a life giver, you're living in your own awareness. The key is to move the bloodstream by moving your body.

Nutrients are brought to the cell through the blood, and a key element in this process is to keep the blood oxygenated. When it receives the nutrients, the cell is stimulated and vibrates. As it vibrates, it becomes healthy. As it vibrates and becomes healthy, it attracts and draws to itself new vibration, new health, and the cell will divide and make another one and divide again and again. You are stimulating the cell into movement. Exercise brings more air into the lungs and when you get more oxygen into the body, the blood is cleaned up and able to effectively deliver nutrients to the cells.

The cell level is energized through clean blood and good oxygen. That's what brings life and vitality. When that is not happening, we get sluggish, lethargic, and we start dying. When we move our body, we raise its vibration. The blood is circulating as the muscles are being stretched and contracted and the bones are being strengthened. The lymph fluid moving through the body can more efficiently do its job of removing waste. More oxygen is getting into the cells, and we are better able to utilize our nutrition.

If you want your body to be cleaner and function better, exercise. It's worth the effort to do it. When you've disciplined your inner process, your outer process starts to flow naturally. So don't exercise just for your body. Exercise for the inner discipline. Once the inner discipline appears, you'll reduce your food consumption, and you'll also find that you will cut down on a lot of bad habits. There's no struggle because you're disciplined.

Moving our bodies also helps balance our emotional state, assists us in reducing stress, and generally brings forward more positive energy and enthusiasm. We are also able to better direct our mind into holding thoughts of what we want more of. Stretching is also a good way to move your body. It detoxifies the blood, moves the lymph through the system, and when done consciously can release restricted patterns of consciousness.

*The cell level is energized through clean blood and good oxygen. That's what brings life and vitality. When that is not happening, we get sluggish, lethargic, and we start dying. When we move our body, we raise its vibration.*

While part of the sympathetic nervous system's function is to get us moving, the parasympathetic nervous system is there to gently put the brakes on. It calms things down. So if you are breathing rapidly in your chest from panic or excitement (a sympathetic system response), by breathing into your belly, you will trigger the parasympathetic nervous system, and you will start to slow down and start moving into a relaxed state.

Since you now know how healthy relaxation is for you (see Principle #4), there is great practicality in understanding and getting a handle on the stress response by becoming more aware of what is happening inside you, in your body, your mind, your imagination, and your emotions. Through positive self-talk, aware breathing, and holding in your mind what you want more of, you can move through life in a more relaxed state, having more energy and enjoying better health.

The calming effects of meditation can also be very helpful in triggering the parasympathetic nervous system and slowing us down. Herbert Benson's mind/body program at Harvard University pioneered the treating of many types of stress-related disorders by teaching patients to meditate. One of the most important yoga poses is Savasana, the corpse pose. This is simply lying down and, perhaps not so simply, completely relaxing.

The most critical thing you can do to recover from being over-stressed is to rest well and get sufficient sleep. This assists the body to clean out the accumulated toxins and start the repair process. The ancient Greeks had temples dedicated to healing where people with sickness came just to rest. That's where we get the phrase, "sleeping it off."

# Less Sugar

I was eating bad stuff. Lots of sugar and carbs, junk food
all the time. It makes you very irritated.

*Avril Lavigne*

There are three types of foods—carbohydrates, proteins, and fats.
All foods fall under one or more of these three categories, and
many foods are made up of all of them in varying proportions.
Many people wonder which category vegetables fit into, and
the surprising answer is that vegetables are carbohydrates. It's
surprising because sugar is also a carbohydrate. Nothing could
seem further apart from a bowl of broccoli than a bowl of sugar,
yet both are in the same food category. This is because the body
breaks down both broccoli and sugar into glucose, which then can
be used for the body's energy needs. There is a large difference in
their taste, the speed with which they get absorbed into the body,
their nutritional value, and their fiber content, but they are both
carbohydrates that eventually end up as glucose.

Within the carbohydrate food category, there are simple
carbohydrates and complex carbohydrates. The simple carbohydrates include sugar and white flour, in other words most of
the desserts you eat. Typically, these foods have little nutritional
value, are high in calories, and are digested quickly causing the
blood sugar to spike upwards. This spike is then usually followed
by a quick drop in blood sugar causing a lowering of our energy
level. This is a reason why simple carbohydrate foods, while often
tempting and delicious, don't really satisfy our hunger, and we get
cravings for more sugar shortly after having eaten them.

Complex carbohydrates tend to be far more nutritious.
These are foods like legumes, whole grains, vegetables, and
most fruits. They are loaded with fiber, antioxidants, vitamins,
and minerals. Calorie-for-calorie, complex carbohydrates will
fill you up more and leave you feeling full a lot longer than
simple carbohydrates.

We need a balance of carbohydrates, proteins, and fats to keep us healthy. Carbohydrates provide us with energy and proteins build and repair tissue. The main purpose of fats is to serve as a storage system and as a reserve supply of energy in the body. During periods of low food consumption, the fat reserves in the body can be mobilized and broken down to release energy. Fats are also used in the body's production of some steroids and hormones that help regulate proper growth and maintenance of tissue in the body. Like carbohydrates, not all fats are equal. There are saturated fats and unsaturated fats and everything in between.

*When unhealthy fats are eaten, such as trans-fats, the cell wall's function is compromised. The cell wall is not just a barrier for the cell, it is responsible for letting in what the cell needs and letting go what it no longer needs.*

When unhealthy fats are eaten, such as trans-fats, the cell wall's function is compromised. The cell wall is not just a barrier for the cell, it is responsible for letting in what the cell needs and letting go what it no longer needs. Often, people are unaware that they can make a trans-fat right in their kitchens simply by heating common oils they buy in the store. Only a few oils, such as coconut oil and sunflower oil, can stay chemically stable in high heat. Oils are best eaten without heating; for example, unprocessed olive oil in a salad dressing. Another good oil to eat is one rich in omega-3 fatty acids; this helps make the cell wall sturdy and functional. Many people take in omega-3 fat in the form of flax oil and salmon or cod liver oil.

Protein is necessary for the building and repair of body tissues. Proteins produce enzymes, hormones, and other important substances that the body uses for its healthy maintenance. Proteins also regulate many body processes, such as hydration in the cells, transporting nutrients, and making muscles contract.

A few years ago, it was a popularly held belief that fats were responsible for the obesity that had mushroomed in the western culture. This launched a proliferation of low fat and non-fat foods, to which sugar and high fructose corn syrup were added to make up for the loss of taste due to the removal of fat. It seemed like the perfect solution to the obesity problem, but after a while, it was discovered that people were putting on more weight than ever, and getting sicker.

Current thinking puts the blame for our culture's proliferation of larger and fatter bodies on carbohydrates, which, as we've seen, the body breaks down into sugar (glucose) for energy. (Note: The argument on whether it is fats or carbohydrates that are responsible for the cultural wave of obesity is still going on. The answer? It depends on the person.)

This takes us back to the bowl of sugar and the bowl of broccoli. The consumption of sugar, a simple carbohydrate, instantaneously affects our blood sugar levels because it is already broken down, and there are no buffers such as fiber to slow its absorption. Eating broccoli, a complex carbohydrate, takes a couple of hours to affect the body because it takes time for the cellulose and the digestible and non-digestible fiber to be processed and broken down. In addition, there are far more minerals and vitamins to be absorbed than refined sugar, which has virtually none.

Each of our cells have various receptor sites. The receptor is like an antenna in that it is a means for the cell to receive communication from other parts of the body. Our body wants the glucose out of our blood and put into our cells where it can be used for energy.

A good analogy would be a car. Having gas in the tank does not make the car move. You need the gas to be injected into the cylinders so that it can combust and then move the car. Therefore, we need to get the nutrients from the blood into the cells so that they can be utilized to produce energy.

Insulin is a hormone that is produced in the pancreas when sugar enters the bloodstream. Insulin attaches to the cell receptor, which then instructs the cell to open the doorway through which glucose can enter. In our modern lifestyles where sugar is in abundance and greatly concentrated in our diet, people will often eat a big meal, have a sweet dessert, and then sit in front of a computer or on the couch watching TV for the rest of the evening. There is some energy that is being utilized in these "activities" but very little in comparison to the high amount of calories being put into the body in the form of sugar.

The body has to do something with this surplus of unused sugar, so it stores it. This is where the fat cells come in. They take the sugar and convert it into fat. It is part of the body's survival mechanism. It now has the sugar stored for another time when it needs energy and food is not immediately available.

When the glucose in the blood has been used up, the insulin removes itself from the cell receptor. This lets the fat cell know that, when more energy is needed somewhere in the body, it can now release its stored fat to provide it. The fat cell does this by converting the stored fat into free fatty acids, which are then released out of the cell into the bloodstream to be available to the cells that need it. It's a wonderful system, but it has started to go awry in our current lifestyle where there are lots of carbohydrates immediately available, and with less exercise, there is a lot of sugar being stored compared to what is being released.

Let's take a hypothetical typical daily eating situation. It begins with cereal for breakfast—a high carbohydrate choice. The cereal causes our blood sugar level to quickly rise (spike). This is immediately followed by an increase in insulin, which is released to get the sugar out of the blood and into the cells. (It's imperative for the body to get the glucose out of the blood as quickly as possible in order to maintain the body's health.)

Over the course of the next hour or two after breakfast, the blood sugar level drops fairly rapidly. Insulin levels also drop but at a much slower rate than the blood sugar, causing us to have a situation where we have low blood sugar and high insulin.

With a cup of coffee and a doughnut, or other high carbohydrate food, the blood sugar spikes up again and the insulin levels rise again. Now you have high blood sugar and high insulin. So it goes on throughout the day as we attempt to manage our energy levels. Notice how sugar vacillates between high and low levels while insulin stays high.

What we refer to as high insulin is the fact that the insulin hormone is still attached to the cell receptor, preventing the cell from converting fat into free fatty acids for release into the bloodstream.

Thus the fat builds up in the cell. This is why the current dietary theory is that carbohydrates are mostly responsible for obesity and not the fats themselves—that sugar is the culprit, not fats.

If you find yourself struggling with fatigue, one possibility is that it could be self-induced by virtue of what we discussed above— that sugar raises blood glucose levels so fast that the body has to respond by secreting large amounts of insulin. This cycle creates a huge spike in energy quickly followed by fatigue.

Diabetes is a condition where the quantity of glucose in the blood is too high. This is because the body either does not produce enough insulin, produces no insulin, or has cells that do not respond properly to the insulin the pancreas produces. This results in too much glucose building up in the blood. This excess blood glucose eventually passes out of the body in urine. So, even though the blood has plenty of glucose, the cells are not getting it for their essential energy and growth requirements.

*If you find yourself struggling with fatigue, one possibility is that it could be self-induced by virtue of what we discussed above—that sugar raises blood glucose levels so fast that the body has to respond by secreting large amounts of insulin.*

A healthy pancreas adjusts the amount of insulin based on the level of glucose. But if you have diabetes, this process breaks down, and blood sugar levels become too high. People with Type I diabetes are completely unable to produce insulin. People with Type II diabetes can produce insulin, but their cells don't respond to it. In either case, the glucose can't move into the cells, and blood glucose levels can become high. Over time, these high glucose levels can cause serious complications.

Pre-diabetes is where the cells in your body are becoming resistant to insulin or your pancreas is not producing as much insulin as required. Your blood glucose levels are higher than normal but not high enough to be called diabetes. A diagnosis of pre-diabetes is a warning sign that diabetes could develop later. The good news is that by making lifestyle changes, you can prevent the development of Type II diabetes through losing weight, better nutrition, exercise, and adequate rest and sleep.

To see how ubiquitous sugar is in our diet, take a moment to understand the words in our vocabulary that relate to sugar. The prefix "gly-" means "sugar." The suffix "-emia" means "in the blood."

Thus, glycemia means "sugar in the blood." The prefix "hypo-" means "low" and "hyper-" means "over or above," so hypoglycemia is a chronic low blood sugar condition. The suffix "–ose" also means "sugar," so lactose, found in milk, means "milk sugar."

Recognizing all that we have spoken about in this chapter, a few years ago scientists, in order to calibrate which foods spiked blood sugar more than others, developed a "Glycemic Index." Some specialized diets choose only low glycemic foods to regulate blood sugar.

Another situation that arises from high blood sugar is called glycation. In short, glycation is a scientific term for what happens when sugars, such as fructose or glucose, combine with proteins or lipid molecules. More simply put, glycation is the process bakers and cooks refer to as browning or caramelization. While crisp French fries and grilled meats may be tasty, the health effects are questionable. When we brown or caramelize a food, we are glycating it. This caramelization actually happens to us, in our bodies, as we age. From a so-called "anti-aging" perspective, this is not a healthy thing as in a high sugar environment, our cells get sugar-coated. Instead of being in their healthy, slippery state—being able to move over and under each other with freedom and ease—they start sticking to each other, making the cell less efficient and causing a breakdown in the tissue and other health problems.

Sugars are added to many of our foods specifically to enhance this browning effect. Something called Advanced Glycation End Products (AGEs) are formed when sugars are cooked with proteins and fats. Once absorbed by your body, AGEs are well known inflammatory and disease-causing compounds. AGEs have been implicated in many age-related chronic diseases such as: Type II diabetes, cardiovascular disease, Alzheimer's disease, cancer, neuropathy, and the list goes on.

It is also helpful to familiarize yourself with what are called free radicals. Free radicals are highly unstable molecules that interact quickly and aggressively with other molecules in our bodies to create abnormal cells. Oxidative stress occurs when the available supply of the body's antioxidants is insufficient to handle and neutralize free radicals of different types. The result is cell damage that can then result in cellular mutations, tissue breakdown, inflammation, and immune system compromise.

Glycated proteins are estimated to generate 50 times more free radicals than non-glycated proteins. Perhaps you are seeing why many health practitioners say that our bodies were not designed to handle the simple sugars that find their way into our diets. Fortunately, there are certain nutrients that may serve as glycation inhibitors. Among those that have shown promising results are cinnamon, black pepper, ginger, cumin, and green tea.

Scientists have also discovered that alpha lipoic acid can arrest the glycation process. Additionally, it has been discovered that N-acetyl-cysteine (NAC) slows the glycation process and the flavanoids found in fruits, vegetables, and whole grains have been found to reduce the glycation of hemoglobin, the protein responsible for oxygen transport in the blood. This is all research that is still evolving so if it is something that you find relevant for your own health, it is best to check it out with your health-care practitioner.

While glycation, AGEs, and free radicals appear to be among leading factors that initiate many of our age-related diseases, we have the ability to avoid being a victim to these processes. It is really a choice on our part. If you have watched anyone in their later years suffer from one of the debilitating health problems we mentioned earlier, and you thought to yourself that you wanted a different path, you have that option. However, it is not about making that decision for just a single day. It requires a commitment to a lifestyle change. That change includes replacing simple sugars and (glycated) deep fried foods with healthy, nutritious foods. While it is easy to be tempted from time to time by the convenience of fast foods, with the abundance these days of fresh organic foods and high quality food supplements, combined with good rest and exercise, we have the tools we need to live long and healthy lives.

As covered in the previous chapter, cortisol also plays an important role. Cortisol, which controls blood sugar, should remain low at night. Adrenal glands make cortisol. If the adrenal glands become malfunctioning through constant stress, the result is an inability to smoothly orchestrate cellular insulin and glucose transportation through the body. This can cause depression and anxiety among other health issues. A too-high sugar condition in the blood causes spikes of cortisol trying to control the sugar and insulin. Cortisol spikes are like little jolts of adrenaline and caffeine, which are not conducive to a good night's rest.

When it comes to regulating blood sugar, proteins also play a vitally important role in addition to their function of building and repairing tissue. By reducing our intake of simple carbohydrates, such as sugar and refined flour, and replacing them with more complex carbohydrates like vegetables, and by adding more protein to the mix—eggs, nuts, meat, fish, etc.—the blood sugar won't tend to spike, and we'll have a lower and more steady blood sugar level, with a lower insulin level to match. With lower insulin the free fatty acids will be able to be released from the fat cell into the bloodstream, and the body will be able to function more efficiently.

*By reducing our intake of simple carbohydrates, such as sugar and refined flour, and replacing them with more complex carbohydrates like vegetables, and by adding more protein to the mix—eggs, nuts, meat, fish, etc.—the blood sugar won't tend to spike, and we'll have a lower and more steady blood sugar level, with a lower insulin level to match.*

Note that there are some foods that are natural blood sugar stabilizers, such as cinnamon, black pepper, coconut oil, and all foods high in fiber, because this slows the metabolism of the sugar into the bloodstream.

It is not very practical, or desirable, to eliminate all sugar in your diet. However, it is certainly possible for most of us to reduce the amount of sugar we consume. Keep in mind that by some estimates the average American consumes roughly 24 teaspoons of sugar daily. So it's advisable, as a first and easy step, to reduce the simple sugars in your diet. You probably don't need to eat as much bread, pasta, and pie as you do. As you cut down on the excess of these refined carbohydrates, you will undoubtedly be assisting your cells to perform more efficiently, and thus you will be healthier.

Also, do your best to reduce AGE-laden foods by limiting browned or charred foods in your diet, such as well-done meats, fried eggs, and particularly deep fried foods. You can avoid AGEs by boiling, poaching, steaming, and baking foods to keep AGEs from forming. The same foods prepared with water as a cooking medium, instead of oil or over a grill, have been found to greatly reduce these aging compounds. If you eat a lot of carbohydrates before you go to bed, during the night you will be storing fat with high insulin levels instead of releasing free fatty acids.

All this information says that one of the best ways to tackle obesity and the onset of diabetes is to eat less sugar and move our bodies more. Are you willing to make those changes that will make you healthier? If yes, what small change can you make that you can be consistent with?

# Less Acid

The terrain is everything.

*Claude Bernard*

Bernard was right, the germ is nothing—the milieu
(the environment within) is everything.

*Louis Pasteur (on his deathbed)*

High acidity is the most common acid-alkaline balance
problem. When the body's mineral reserves are depleted,
the body "borrows" minerals from whatever source it
can. This usually means that minerals are borrowed
from bones and vital organs. Over time this weakens the
organs and muscles.

*David Murphy, Ph.D.*

If we live and die at the cell level, how can we create an environment
in our bodies in which our cells can flourish and regenerate? The
answer is a multifaceted one, but one of the more critical of those
facets is the acid/alkaline balance of the body. There are many
varying opinions on this subject, but there are some general trends
that are clear and that you can utilize for your benefit.

We've all heard that we should do things in moderation, and
indeed, it is good advice when it comes to our bodies. The reason
that extremes of anything tend to not be good for the body is
because the body's natural direction is towards health and balance
and homeostasis. Homeostasis is a stable equilibrium that the
body strives to maintain so that the body's systems can function
optimally. No example of homeostasis is more apparent than in
the acid/alkaline balance within the body. The body essentially
functions better in a slightly alkaline environment.

We can measure whether something is acid or alkaline by its "pH" factor (pH means potential of hydrogen). A substance that is seen as being pH neutral is one that shows a reading of 7.0 pH. That's the level of natural, pure water. A lower reading than 7.0 indicates that the substance is acid. A higher reading than 7.0 pH indicates that it is alkaline. Blood, for example, is slightly alkaline, and our cells are also slightly alkaline.

Although a slightly alkaline environment is a healthier environment for the body, through our day-to-day lifestyles, we tend to create more of an acid environment, not only through the food we eat but also through our negative thoughts, emotional reactivity, and poor breathing habits.

When we think of the word acid, we usually think of corrosion. If we pour acid on something, it usually begins the process of breaking it down. It's the same with the body—if it is overly acidic for an extended period of time, cell tissue starts to show premature wear and tear.

It can be fun to get away with our bad habits when we are young, but as we get older, we start to pay for them. A good example is eating fast food. From observation we can deduce that consuming fast food is detrimental to health, because the populations of many countries that adopt an American fast food diet get health problems, such as heart disease and obesity, within a short time.

When we eat a cheeseburger, french fries, and a cola, we are flooding our bodies with acidity, because those particular foods are very acid producing. The body being the brilliant mechanism that it is, in striving for homeostasis, needs to balance this acid influx as soon as it hits the bloodstream. An immediate reaction is critical because the blood has a narrow band in which it can properly function—7.35-7.45 pH. If the blood becomes acid at 6.9 pH, the body can start to go into a coma.

In order to balance the acid entering the system, the body has a built-in buffering system within the blood itself to counteract it. This buffering system has two primary organs involved in the

*Although a slightly alkaline environment is a healthier environment for the body, through our day-to-day lifestyles, we tend to create more of an acid environment, not only through the food we eat but also through our negative thoughts, emotional reactivity, and poor breathing habits.*

moment to moment adjustment of the body's pH: the lungs and the kidneys, releasing carbon dioxide from the lungs and various acids through the kidneys.

The bones also contain alkalizing minerals. Indeed, 85% of our body's acid-buffering capacity is contained in the calcium carbonate of bone. Ideally, we want to manage our pH through diet, stress management, and allowing the lung and kidney functions to do their jobs so we can preserve our bone mass. Otherwise, the body will draw minerals, such as calcium carbonate, sodium, magnesium, and potassium, from the bones when our system becomes too acidic. These minerals have an electric charge and are called electrolytes. They are dynamically involved in maintaining the acid/alkaline balance in the body. In an extended acid state, more and more minerals are drawn from the bones, and this is a suspected cause of osteoporosis.

When we put food in our mouth, in order for the starches to be broken down, our saliva is slightly acid. However, our mouth does not have sufficient acid to break down meat, which is broken down in the stomach with hydrochloric acid. The proper place in our bodies to be acid is in the stomach. However, when we get older we tend not to produce enough acid to break down proteins and kill off unwanted bacteria. With less acid in the stomach breaking down the food, our ability to absorb nutrients decreases. When we feel heartburn and take an antacid we are actually neutralizing the acid in our stomach and compromising its function.

As the food moves down the digestive tract to the small intestine, we don't want the hydrochloric acid to come in contact with the surface tissues of the intestines, so bile is produced by the gall bladder while bicarbonate is produced by the pancreas in order to balance the acid. These substances go about alkalizing, as well as breaking down and aiding in the assimilation of our food. (By the time our food is just a few inches into the small bowel, it is back to neutral pH.) In addition, the lungs provide oxygen, and release carbon dioxide, another alkalizing process. The kidneys also produce their own buffers, selectively excreting acids into the urine, and adjusting electrolytes as the blood passes through them.

There are ways to measure the acid/alkaline balance in the body. Taking a strip of pH paper and putting it in your urine stream can measure the acidity that is being excreted by the kidneys. The pH paper, which can be bought at a pharmacy, changes color, and the shade will indicate the pH level of the urine. The pH of the saliva can also be measured in a similar way by putting the pH paper in your mouth. However, the most critical pH is that of the blood and that requires a more sophisticated testing at a medical facility.

*Having an excess of sugar in our bodies, through eating simple carbohydrates, is another way that we create an acid condition in the body, especially high fructose corn syrup, which increases uric acid, among other effects.*

What are the most common consequences of an over acid body? For one thing there will be a tendency to get colds. Heartburn is another consequence. A common over-the-counter remedy for heartburn is Alka-Seltzer—alkalizing seltzer, which is primarily made up of bicarbonate of soda. I have recommended for years a simple combination of baking soda (bicarbonate of soda) and cream of tartar. You can take up to a teaspoon of each in a glass of water, and it will greatly assist the body to come into its acid/alkaline balance. It can also be effective in clearing radiation from the environment in the body (which is in higher concentrations after a rainstorm) and can assist in alleviating cold symptoms.

Having an excess of sugar in our bodies, through eating simple carbohydrates, is another way that we create an acid condition in the body, especially high fructose corn syrup, which increases uric acid, among other effects. Many people get colds at holiday times as people tend to overdo pies, sweets, and other dessert foods, plus there is the stress that tends to go with visiting family and traveling long distances to see them.

The body fighting off allergies will also create an acid condition. It is important to watch if eating certain foods causes you to have adverse reactions so you can avoid putting them in your system. Oftentimes, it is necessary to track in a daily journal what you are eating so you are more consciously aware of what foods are working for you and what foods are making you sick. If the immune system is occupied with an allergy to a food that you are putting in your system, then it has less attention and energy to give to invading foreign bacteria and viruses, setting up an inflammatory reactive state in the body, and contributing to an acidic internal environment.

Other symptoms of an over-acid body are sore and aching joints. If you wake up in the morning and your joints are stiff, or you have a backache, it may be an indication that your system is too acidic. (There can be other reasons for this such as the need to hydrate the body so be sure to check with your healthcare professional.) An acid environment in the body will start to break down the body's tissues. Modern medicine has established that when the blood becomes over acidic, it can create an environment for cancer.

*If it's accurate that cancer can't proliferate in an alkaline environment, and that the regeneration and repair of cells takes place in an alkaline environment, it obviously behooves us to know how we can alkalize our bodies.*

If it's accurate that cancer can't proliferate in an alkaline environment, and that the regeneration and repair of cells takes place in an alkaline environment, it obviously behooves us to know how we can alkalize our bodies. We can start with our breath as the lungs have a vital role because oxygen is an alkalizing agent. In fact, the function of the lungs is probably 50% to 70% of our alkalizing process. When we inhale, we take in alkalizing oxygen, and when we exhale, we release acidic carbon dioxide. That is not to say that carbon dioxide is entirely bad; it is actually essential to a functioning body. But if we're over acid, we can help restore balance by some good, deep breathing—ideally in an oxygen-rich environment.

As we've discussed, the stress response creates a toxic, acid response in the body, so if we can activate our parasympathetic nervous system through the process of diaphragmatic breathing, then we will tend towards being more alkaline the more we relax. Meditation, spiritual exercises, deep breathing, and relaxation are all part of creating a healthy, slightly alkaline terrain (inner environment) for the cells to thrive and regenerate.

Nutrition, as always, is very important too. There are alkalizing foods and acid-forming foods. Since there are differing views on this, it's best to do your own research on the Internet or consult with your healthcare practitioner. But it's fair to say that vegetables, particularly green leafy vegetables, are alkalizing for the body. So are foods that have a high potassium, calcium, or sodium mineral content.

To once again emphasize this: Breathe. Oxygen is required for life. You can live forty days without food and ten days without water, but you can live only four minutes without air.

*Cells have the ability to regenerate and duplicate exact replicas of themselves many times without any deterioration.*

Cells have the ability to regenerate and duplicate exact replicas of themselves many times without any deterioration. There is accuracy in the quote that "the terrain is everything" as it is invariably the environment that we have created within our bodies (not only physically but also what we do in our minds and with our emotions) that is the main factor in our longevity. Poor diet and pollution are degenerative factors, but negative thoughts and emotions also very much contribute to the body's acid content.

Our aging and the wearing down of our bodies essentially come down to this inner terrain that all of us live in. We create an acid environment for ourselves through the lifestyle we lead, the foods we eat, the toxins we don't eliminate, the negative images we hold, the judgments we make, etc. Fortunately, it is within our ability to choose to create a slightly alkaline one. Silent inflammation in combination with an internal over-acid environment contribute to accelerating aging and chronic disease.

A doctor friend of mine, working in Los Angeles, said that in his 30-year practice, he had only seen two new patients who had healthy inner terrains from measuring their pH. One had been in Hawaii for two weeks, in Tahiti for two more weeks, and had exercised and rested a lot in that oxygen-rich environment. The other one was a yoga teacher who was specialized in Pranayama—the branch of yoga that focuses on breathing. Those examples are certainly a testament to the alkalizing effects of good breathing and getting oxygen into our systems.

A lot of techniques that we are giving in this book go in the direction of alkalizing the body, for example, the techniques of forgiveness and meditation. Although research has not been done on this specifically, there is plenty of anecdotal evidence that gratitude is alkalizing and that laughter is too.

It's no accident that "laughter is the best medicine" and that humor begins with "HU" *(see page 179)*. So to alkalize—HU more. An old Irish proverb says, "A good laugh and a long sleep are the best cures in the doctor's book."

We can get so serious about health and illness, when healing can so often be found in laughter. Don't forget to love yourself and laugh at yourself. In the midst of the most terrible, wrenching, insidious thing going on inside of you, laugh. That's the time you need to laugh the most. You have to get something to counterbalance the awful thing you have conjured up, and laughter starts to balance it out.

If you don't feel like laughing, that's the time to laugh. You can release yourself from the weight of the past through laughter. Even in your daily life, if you can laugh instead of taking umbrage at some of the things that people say or do, then you are already free at that moment and the situation can't hang on to you.

As you go through your day, keep dropping away anything that is not the peace that you want. Laugh, have fun, breathe, and be joyful. Humor and laughter are good for the immune system and good for alkalizing the system.

Causes and Cures of Disease

I've titled this chapter *Causes and Cures of Disease*, because most of us are very concerned about why we get sick. Here I've outlined the causes of illness and disease that I have found; but more importantly, I also discuss the cures I've found. The cure is always found spiritually. On the way to spiritual healing, you may need to see medical doctors or some qualified person trained in the psychological approach. If you are able to get to the essence of what I'm talking about here, you'll be able to have a greater understanding of what has bothered you in your life and how you can change it. This is not about demanding that others change. My work points all responsibility for your life back to you.

Most of us have empowered other people to have control over our lives. We have given the responsibility for our lives over to spouses, doctors, educational institutions, various government offices, etc. In fact, we'll empower anyone who we think has more know-how than we do.

Most of our diseases come out of our emotions. Everyone in this world has emotions. What we do with the emotions is how we take charge of our lives. What the emotions do to us is how we let life take charge of us. No one wants to be a victim, and in this section, I hope to take away your victim consciousness. For each reason you have for feeling like a victim, I have an alternative approach in this chapter for you to change it.

The workings of the body are enormously complex, and if you are not a scientist or a doctor, they can seem rather overwhelming. However, as we have seen, everything is energy. So from an energetic standpoint, we can deal much more effectively and practically with the body by realizing that, as energy beings, we are either expanding or contracting. There is a healthy element to this in terms of growth, but also an unhealthy element when we become stuck in our contraction. That stuckness is where disease enters.

There's some very good news in all of this. We can, through being aware of where we are stuck, choose to expand and thereby regain our health and vitality. In other words, inherent within the disease is the cure. I think we have all heard that the cure for the sting of the stinging nettle, the dock leaf, is always growing close by. But what is little known is that the antidote is within the stem of the stinging nettle itself. This latter point is the metaphor we are after, for while we can go outside of us for a "cure," the true cure is found inside each of us.

Sometimes it may not be wise to be in such a hurry to get a cure. Sometimes it can be best to sit with the dis-ease, see what it is, and see what our responsibility is in creating it. If we take a pill and our symptoms go away, that doesn't mean the situation has been completed. It can resurface again.

Get out of the idea that there is something "wrong" with you if you have an illness, dis-ease, or a physical, mental, or emotional difficulty. It would be more correct to say you are being presented with a learning opportunity—a gift, in fact. So instead of judging yourself, start to take responsibility for the causes of your dis-ease. Only by taking responsibility for the cause can you receive the gift of the lesson and, by learning the lesson, receive the cure.

The "magic" is in your attitude and your openness. In many ways, it takes a certain ruthlessness to look at your patterns. It takes great courage to see the face of God, but the first step is to see your own "face" clearly and lovingly and without judgment or contraction.

Most of us seek cures before we will acknowledge the causes. Most people are looking for someone to fix them or give them the right pill, yet we can often find the solution by looking at what we are doing, instead of needing to do more. The cures we seek are often a way of our avoiding taking responsibility for the causes. When we listen to ourselves in the correct way, we may realize that the problem is presenting the solution to our healing.

I hope it's clear that it can be very helpful, educational, and healing to look at your illness, dis-ease, or incapacity as a perfect teacher for you. Now, can you be the perfect student? What is there for you to learn? What gift is this situation bringing you?

In looking at these causes and cures, consider what Albert Einstein said: "You cannot solve a problem with the same consciousness that created it." Inherent within that statement is the idea that if what we are doing is not working for us, we need to start doing things differently. Most of us do the same things over and over again, hoping to bring about change. That's not changing anything; that's being crazy.

Some people say, "This can't be changed. It's karmic." It may well be karma (the effect of prior actions). However, hearing that something is karmic is not a reason to give up. I've seen a lot of conditions that were karmic and were subsequently healed by the person bringing their Soul energy into the situation and using that to heal.

The difficulty that most people face when they have a karmic illness of some kind—any karmic situation in fact—is that they have too much evidence that their condition is really bad. To tell them to think positively just doesn't work at all, because as soon as they think positively and something doesn't work, they immediately think negatively again.

However, we can all keep a positive focus. The old metaphysicians used to call it "out-picturing"—to get a picture in our mind that represents health the way we want to experience it. That means getting the picture as strong inside you as if you were looking at a photo in a magazine. It has to have detail in it: the color, the flow, the feeling, which you can then start to put out in front of you as if that image is your body and your consciousness, and you keep moving into that image until it becomes real for you.

You actually enter into this new, healthy body as if you were a spirit in the room seeing a body in full health and walking into it. You picture health and then make the picture become real as you move to it. At the point that happens, you integrate it into yourself.

How do you bring kidneys and other areas of the body back to health? This is where you create your own inner sanctuary. Within that sanctuary you have a Resource Center. You can imagine this

Resource Center as having all the technology you need. There you put an image of your body up on a big screen, and you operate on yourself. Take out the bad organs, joints, etc., and snap in the new ones. This is another way of out-picturing what you want, but you're picturing it deep within yourself.

It is stated in the Bible that as a man thinks, in his heart he becomes *(Proverbs 23:7 NIV)*. Most people know that energy follows thought. Often, our emotions (energy in motion) will calm right down if we change what we are thinking about. What is less known is that thought, for the most part, follows perception. How you perceive, or what you perceive, is the seed for what's going to be around you energetically and thus what's likely to manifest in your life. If you watch or read violent or sex-oriented movies or literature, what you see or read is going to start producing the seed for the energy to follow. If you look at a sunset and take that in, the energy of the beauty of that sunset will also start to form energy fields inside you.

Your perceptions are important. But there's an even easier way to move towards healing, and that's to lift yourself, in the Soul, above the field of action, contact the spiritual energy, the Holy Spirit, and, for your highest good, let it flood and radiate down and disintegrate away from you what you no longer need.

I learned that if I contact this Soul energy, this impulse field of life, and if I just sit and do nothing with it, it starts to move down over me like a shower—in a spiraling, undulating motion. You can sometimes feel a little dizzy as it undulates and moves. It will just pop away any negative thought forms you are holding onto or that are holding onto you.

You can contact this Soul energy field through spiritual exercises, through chanting the "HU" or "ANI-HU." You can also chant the "OM." The OM vibrates in the lower mental part of consciousness, but sometimes that's all you need. Doing this can clear your energy field of those negative forms that could have eventually resulted in illness and disease.

When the negativity clears, you look at people and you see beauty all around because the Soul will impulse down through the lower levels of consciousness and will start to knock away the debris of the negative thinking and thought forms.

Thought forms are undirected and incomplete energy that we put out and get caught in our energy field where they attract negative energy. When you let your Light shine, it just keeps pulling away everything that is not of the Soul impulse. It's released through the Soul energy of the Holy Spirit coming through and moving around you. You let it fall away. If we go into the Soul energy and allow it to impulse down, whatever is in the thought form will be transformed into Light. If you do really have the desire of God in you, it will start the energy of your Soul moving. God is inside in the Soul center and is the only one that can really move and release the thought form.

We get thought forms because we do not put in our mind what we want and the result we want from it. If the negative thought forms are not taken care of, they can get into the physical body, and we may start to have illness and disease. It's very important that we watch what we put in our mind, what we hold in our mind, and the direction we're going with our mind. Now, in reality, there is only one mind. It's the mind of God. But there are many aspects, avenues, and expressions of that one mind, and we're living proof of that.

Our minds are tricky. When we think something, we think it's true. If I could get you to see how wrong and what a fundamental mistake that thinking is, you would be further ahead. In actuality, because you think, you think. What you think may not be true at all.

Are you supposed to believe everything that's being said here? No, you're supposed to be open to your own Soul's impulse. Have you ever found out that when you start to question the good feeling you have, it starts to go away? That's the thought forms building up again. When you start to enjoy the process of life, the mind starts to move into joyful thinking patterns. We start to play inspirational music and to sing or hum along or move our bodies with it. We read uplifting poetry and look at beautiful art. When we find those things that bring joy and happiness to our mind and emotions, the heart opens and the dis-ease of the body begins to peel away.

In this chapter, I've given you several pathways to better health. None of them are necessarily easy or fast; otherwise, we'd all be doing them, and we would have very few health problems on the planet. If you can approach these pathways with the attitude of being joyful, regardless of the outcome, you can't lose.

I'd like you to look at each one of these causes of disease as though that is the only thing that you have in your life. When you read the cause, see if there is a place inside you that responds to that word and allow it to come forward so that you can see and know what it feels like.

When I give the cure, get the essence of the cure and put it on the diseased word and transmute the diseased word into the health word. It may assist you to do this with a symbolic hand gesture of placing one palm on top of the other. Some people reading this are going to do it instantly. Some, who think they have an incurable illness, may take longer. But I would like everybody to do this. No excuses.

There is much more I could have said about each cause and cure. I never attempt to give anyone the final word on anything. You would no longer grow. Instead, I hang the carrot out in front of you so that you can explore more for yourself and find the spiritual being that you are.

Choose a relaxed time to look deeply at these causes and cures. The *Things to act upon and questions to ask yourself and ponder* are designed to call forward from within you any restrictions, constrictions, or imbalances so they can be balanced and healed. If you get clear information and knowledge about your situation, you may, through awareness, through forgiveness, and through the Light, no longer need the experience of the dis-ease. Now that would be a great completion!

# Cause

## 1

---

### RESTRAINT

Restraint means that we want to do something, but we are not sure how it will turn out. In not knowing how it will turn out, we tend to constrict ourselves inside. Restraint is where we hold ourselves back from living our life fully and where we won't allow ourselves to move forward because the thoughts and beliefs we are holding onto block us from looking and perceiving accurately. When we restrain ourselves, we go out of balance.

*Not trusting ourselves leads to our not being able to make up our minds and proceed with purpose.*

Part of this process is thinking that if we make a mistake, it will be a disaster. But the opportunity in making a mistake is, when we know what the mistake is, we can correct it. When we correct it, we're wiser than before we made the mistake. A mistake shows you what we can learn. Do not be afraid of mistakes. This planet is full of them.

When we have restraint, we do not breathe deeply. We breathe in a shallow way, and we do not use our lungs to their full capacity. Thus, we do not oxygenate the blood as well as we can and the nutrients don't get into the cells in an optimal way. The result is that what goes with restraint are aches and pains. When we have aches and pains, we have an excuse not to do what needs to get done.

What is it that restrains us? Often it's other people's opinions or our thoughts that we won't have enough money to do what we want and, as we've seen, our fear of making a mistake. This leads to our not following through, which in turn leads to our not trusting ourselves. Not trusting ourselves leads to our not being able to make up our minds and proceed with purpose.

Can you now understand how restraint can be a disease? It's not a disease in the medical or pathological sense; it's a disease of consciousness.

Things to act upon and questions to ask yourself and ponder:

1)  How do you hold yourself back?

2)  Recall a time when you have done this.

3)  What beliefs and thoughts are you holding that limit you?

4)  What mistake are you afraid of making?

5)  What mistake have you made that you have not let go of?

6)  In what ways may you be holding concern about others' opinions of you?

7)  Describe your self-talk with any of (1) to (6) above.

8)  Now describe how you can proceed with purpose.

9)  When you hold yourself back, in which part of your body do you feel tightness or imbalance?

10) Forgive yourself for any judgments you are holding (see *Appendix: Forgiveness* page 249).

11) Gently exhale and now take in a deep breath. Start to find ways to use your lungs to their capacity in order to oxygenate the cells.

12) Place the Light in and through you (see *Healing Light* page 161).

# Cure

## 1

---

### LOVE

The cure for restraint is to love what you're doing. When the loving is present and alive inside you, you handle things beautifully. So when you're going to do something and you're not sure of the outcome, love yourself while you're doing it. You don't have to love the outcome because you may not know the outcome, but you can love yourself all the way to the outcome. Then, when you get to the end, you will have love. You will also have success.

*Feel the love come into your body, and then start putting one foot in front of the other.*

Success can be blocked by the disease called restraint. So anytime you feel restraint, for whatever the reason, start looking inside and feeling the love. Don't get preoccupied by what the worries you are carrying in your mind and emotions are about. Feel the love come into your body, and then start putting one foot in front of the other. Literally. It's very simple, and it will not be long until you'll be at your goal.

Some of you will say, "I can't walk that far; it's two miles." It's going to be two miles if you do it tomorrow, next week, or next year. If you start now, you'll be on your way. It is the thought of restraint and the feeling of constriction that stops you from going forward.

Action is the keynote to releasing restraint. You love yourself enough to get the seat of your pants off the seat of the chair and get going. Unless, of course, you're a writer, in which case get the seat of your pants on the seat of the chair—and get going.

You can always break down projects into simple steps and set short range goals. There's a simple next step to everything, and that simple step can always be taken in a relaxed way. So, from now on, no excuses. Move forward. Regardless of your ache or pain, get up and go do what you want or need to do anyway. And, love yourself along the way.

1) What action do you need to take today?
   (Say the first thought that comes to mind.)

2) As you mock-up doing what you just described,
   do you feel this action releasing your restraint?

3) If you answered no to (2), what action can you
   take that would release your restraint?

4) If the action cannot be taken all at once, what is the
   smallest step you can take—a microscopic movement
   towards what you need to do?

5) What image can you hold to inspire you to act?

6) What do you need to say to yourself to get you moving—
   your positive self-talk?

7) How do you hold back your love from yourself?

8) What needs to be loved, right now?

9) Put your hands over your heart and feel the loving going
   in and through your body.

10) Now get the essence of love inside you and, as an inner
    process, put it on or over the cause, restraint. You can also
    do this with a hand gesture, placing one palm on top of
    the other. Allow the cause of dis-ease to be transmuted
    into the cure of health and well-being. You can ask for the
    assistance of the Light in this process and remember also
    to always ask for the highest good.

11) Describe how you are feeling inside.

12) What have you learned?

# Cause
# 2

_____

## FEAR

There is no real source of fear, but there is a real feeling of fear. If fear has no real source, and it's a real feeling, where is this fear coming from? We are creating it. Restraint works to produce the feeling of fear. Your feelings about something are what you are doing inside. It's your energy following your thoughts or perceptions.

We can experience things that do not have a real source to them. But the mind and the emotions don't know that and can live in fear and amplify it using that as the reason not to perform in this world. Your internal dialogue will sound something like, "What will they think of me? What if I fail? What if I'm no good? What if I make a mistake?"

1) What do you feel fearful of?

2) What other emotions surface when you answer (1)?
   (Describe them in terms of your self-talk.)

3) What thoughts do you hold that keep the fear in place?
   (Describe them in terms of your self-talk.)

4) Take ten seconds or so to focus on your breath and only
   your breath—its rising and falling.

5) Take in the awareness that it is only your thoughts, and the
   emotions they surface, that create the fear.

6) What pictures or images can you hold in your mind that
   you want more of?

7) Forgive yourself for any judgments you have been holding.

8) Close your eyes and connect with your divinity. Let your
   Soul energy impulse down and dissolve the thought form
   and emotional energy of fear you have been holding.

# Cure

## 2

### EMPATHY

The cure for fear is empathy. Empathy is a form of understanding. Fear can be a statement of "I'm alone, I'm different, and there's nobody else around." The opposite of that is empathy. When you move into the feeling level with somebody who has fear and come into contact with them in that way, to be as one with them in empathy produces such an environment of understanding that fear cannot abide in it.

*In this empathetic process, no one loses their identity, the preciousness of the Soul.*

If you see somebody experiencing fear, it's no use saying to them, "Don't worry, there is no fear," because they feel fear. So they don't believe you. They think you don't understand. But if you say, "I understand you're experiencing fear. Where is the fear coming from?" They will say, "It's coming from my mind. It's about my thoughts about what has happened to me." It could be an unfortunate love affair or losing a job. Then you can say, "I understand. You can use the fear as a reason not to go on with your life, or you can reach inside you to the place where you find love, grab the strength from that love, put it through empathy, and change the fear to caution."

It is only through empathy that it is possible to step into another person's shoes without displacing that person or without forcing yourself upon them and restricting and controlling them. In this empathetic process, no one loses their identity, the preciousness of the Soul.

God is pouring forth the Spirit into these days that we are living in now. And even though we may see starvation, floods, wars, and countries going bankrupt, we will know the law of empathy, for empathy is a spiritual law. If we don't know starvation, and we have no empathy, it will be brought to us to experience it. God bless those who can move to the law of empathy, for you sidestep the lessons that would be presented to you otherwise.

**Things to act upon and questions to ask yourself and ponder:**

1) Forgive yourself for any separation you have created between yourself and your loving, between yourself and others, and between yourself and God.

2) Say to yourself, "I forgive myself for forgetting that I am divine."

3) Soften any hardness you may be carrying. Open your heart, and reach out to someone you know in person, by phone, or over the Internet, in a loving, caring, and empathetic way.

4) Observe what happens inside you to any fear you may have been carrying at even the thought of doing (3) above.

5) Now get the essence of empathy inside you, and as an inner process, put it on or over the cause, fear. You can also do this with a hand gesture, placing one palm on top of the other. Allow the cause of dis-ease to be transmuted into the cure of health and well-being. You can ask for the assistance of the Light in this process and remember also to always ask for the highest good.

6) Describe how you are feeling inside.

7) What have you learned?

# Cause

# 3

---

## RESTLESSNESS

It seems strange to call restlessness a disease but let's look at some of the ways restlessness works.

*Restlessness is all internal—it's all inside of us.*

Restlessness is where you want to get an educational degree, but you are so restless you can't sit and study because you've got other things that you must do. Or you want to go see the doctor for a check-up, but you don't go because you are too restless to wait in the waiting room.

A husband that is restless with his wife develops a roving eye, and so he goes to find rest somewhere else. If he finds rest somewhere else, then he starts to have fear and restraint towards his wife. If she's paying attention, she will know right away he's done something out of line. It's the same process when a wife is restless with her husband.

Restlessness is also the feeling of wanting to do something but not knowing what to do. Restlessness is all internal—it's all inside of us. As soon as we get up and start moving, the restlessness starts to disappear as the energy is directed.

Restlessness on the job means you are not being challenged in your work. Instead of looking for another job, you can go to your employer and tell them that you feel you need to learn more, that you need to grow, and that you would like to grow with the company. If they liked you enough to hire you, they'll likely want to keep you.

Of course, you may fear that you'll get a job you can't handle, so then you'll feel restraint in asking. Then you won't get the money you want. So then you have more restlessness because you want things in life and you don't have the money. Can you see how these causes work together?

Things to act upon and questions to ask yourself and ponder:

1) What are you restless or dissatisfied about?

2) What do you need to move on in your life?

3) What's the smallest step (microscopic movement) you can take to get you going in a positive direction?

4) What do you want in your life that is on purpose for you?

5) What is stopping you from getting what you answered in (4) above?

6) Forgive yourself for whatever is coming forward for you.

# Cure
# 3

---

## PEACE

The cure for restlessness is peace. We all have an inner war going on—not the war out there among nations or different groups of people, but the war between our mind and our emotions. The war of the emotions is wanting to do something and the mind is saying, "But I can't do that. I'm not trained." Every doctor and every dentist was not trained before they became a doctor or a dentist. Every secretary wasn't born typing. Ballet dancers were not born with ballet shoes on. We can all learn new things all the time. Learning can also mean dropping things that are no longer working for us.

*This peace is a balance between the mind (the thought) and the emotional feeling, so that they are in harmony and balance.*

There is peace inside where the mind and the emotions match, and they have something physically they can move on. Keep this in mind when going towards something you want, like a new job or relationship. This peace is a balance between the mind (the thought) and the emotional feeling, so that they are in harmony and balance. In other words, they are going in the same direction. Often we desire to do one thing, but our mind says that our parents (or our wife or husband) won't like that. So we feel split inside, and that split is the war I am talking about.

To have just a nice thought and a nice feeling and nothing to do, nothing to physically move on, is being an incurable romantic. An incurable romantic does nothing. They lie around and moan and groan about things that are not going well, thinking about how much better things could be. But they are not doing anything to create the better thing.

If you have a good thought about doing something worthwhile, and you have a feeling that matches it, you have a great start because you will have confidence. Now, to have completion, look at how you can physically do it. If there is not a physical place to do it, put it on hold, but don't stop looking for a way to complete it physically. This is so important for your health and well-being.

To give you an example, many years ago I was traveling in Bogota, Colombia, and was looking for a rechargeable battery I needed for my recording machine. I wanted it—my thought and feelings were matched—but I didn't know where to find it physically. The next day, on a day trip to another town, I walked into a store looking for something else, and there was the rechargeable battery. I couldn't find it in Bogota, so I had to put the thought and feeling aside, but I kept looking. When it showed up, I was complete with it. That's what I'm attempting to convey.

If what you want is not immediately in front of you, do not let that disturb your peace of mind. Just know that it will appear. I knew my battery would appear. I just didn't have time to go all over Bogota looking for it. I put it into that place inside of me that I call "divine ignorance." It knows, but it doesn't tell my mind; nevertheless, it led us down the street into the store where we found the battery.

This peace is quieting the body, emotions, and mind and knowing there's a higher force running you. Most of the time when we have a disease, we are so focused on its prognosis and its progress and we are so restless that we don't give ourselves a chance to be calm and quiet and have peacefulness and let the disease leave.

Meditation assists healing because, while the focus is on something else, the body relaxes its pressure on the diseased part, and this allows the energy to come through and start the healing process. The value of meditation is the peacefulness that comes inside. It is not being inactive; it's that there is no tightness and no war inside you. There's quietness, yet activity.

1) Is there a "war" going on inside you where you feel you want to do something, but you think you can't do it—or you feel you can do it, but think you can't?

2) Describe in detail what's going on.

3) Is there something you can move on physically to bring peace to the situation? If so, describe your next step.

4) The simplest meditation is to focus on the rising and falling of your breath. Take a moment to do that right now.

5) Give yourself permission to let go, to relax into yourself and then into your Self.

6) Let your breath be slow and even.

7) Let your breath go deeper into your body.

8) Feel your cells rejoicing in the peace.

9) Now hold in your mind a picture of something beautiful and peaceful. It could be a scene from nature, a tree or the image of a wave, or it could be a pet or a loved one. The healing colors of nature heal and relax your body. The wave rolls through your body relaxing and energizing it. The pet or a loved one opens your heart, and you allow this love to expand, surround, and sanctify you.

10) Know deep within you that peace is always present.

11) Now get the essence of peace inside you, and as an inner process, put it on or over the cause, restlessness. You can also do this with a hand gesture, placing one palm on top of the other. Allow the cause of dis-ease to be transmuted into the cure of health and well-being. You can ask for the assistance of the Light in this process and remember to always ask for the highest good.

12) Describe how you are now feeling inside.

13) What have you learned?

# Cause
# 4

---

## INDECISION

Indecision takes place when you can't make up your mind, and it may be one of the most severe causes of dis-ease. It's where you are saying: "Should I or shouldn't I?" "I'd like to, but I'm not sure." "It's possible but maybe not." "I love them, but I'm not sure how they feel about me." "I want to but, oh, golly." You go up and down, up and down, attempting to make a decision. You have several good reasons for doing something and one reason for not doing it, and you make that one reason not to more valuable than all the other reasons for you to do it. Maybe it is more valuable, but you must look to see, or you may be using your one reason as an excuse to procrastinate and not complete what needs to be done.

Indecision resides, like all the other causes of dis-ease, inside you. Another example is where you want to hug somebody, but you're afraid they will take it the wrong way. The part of you that is in a loving place says to hug them and another part says that maybe they don't want to be hugged.

The solution for this self-made conundrum is to ask them. If they say, "Not now," there is no reason for you to feel rejected as they may want to wait until another time when they feel more comfortable. Maybe they're having personal problems, and they don't want to be touched just now, or perhaps they have rheumatism, or arthritis, or a headache. Often a hug can cure all of that, but they may not know it.

Generally, people who refuse a genuine, loving hug have the war inside of themselves. They also need love more than other people. If you can't tell who needs what, leave them all alone, or hug them all. And you don't always have to hug a person physically.

A few years ago I was walking with a friend of mine, and he said to me, "I am hugging everyone inside of me." That's the way it works best. We walked into a store together, and although it was very busy, the employees went out of their way to help him. He was amazed because normally the employees weren't that helpful. I wasn't surprised at all. When you are hugging somebody inside, they want to help you. You hug them with your eyes, with your inner radiance. You don't have to even smile. The loving, the radiance of the heart, comes up out of you and it smiles.

*When we don't make a decision, a decision ends up being made for us; it's called a decision by default.*

When we don't make a decision, a decision ends up being made for us; it's called a decision by default. That's worse than your making the decision and making a mistake, because in a decision by default, you're inevitably going to blame somebody else to try to make yourself feel better—and that doesn't work either. If you yourself make the error, you can become empowered by owning it, taking charge of it, correcting it, and then starting to make different choices.

Often in a decision by default, you feel like a victim, "I had nothing to do with this. Why does this happen to me?" When we run this type of stuff inside of us, we're out of balance. We are in a constrained position inside of us.

**Things to act upon and questions to ask yourself and ponder:**

1) What are you undecided about?

2) Think of a recent situation where you felt like a victim. Briefly describe it.

3) Was your answer in (2) a result of indecision (decision by default) or was it a poor choice you made?

4) Forgive yourself for any judgments that surface in answering (3) above.

5) Is there an area of indecision currently in your life that you can make up your mind about right now?

6) Realize that you can empower yourself now by letting go of all blame towards others and yourself and owning and taking responsibility for all your indecisions and all your mistakes.

7) What fresh choice can you make to begin your new life?

# Cure
## 4

---

## STEADFASTNESS

The cure for indecision is steadfastness. Once you have made up your mind, you hold the focus until you are complete. It's not that you make up your mind foolishly; you may sit down and write all the pros and cons of your actions and take it apart, being your own devil's advocate to see if anything negative shows up. Anything you find out of balance, correct it. Then the indecision becomes steadfastness, and people may comment how strong you are. You become a leader, not because you want to be a leader but because you've developed the qualities of leadership.

*Humans can do what no other living being in this world can do, and that is to take conscious, corrective action.*

So the cure is to make up your mind, stick to it, and do it. And if it's wrong, correct it. Humans can do what no other living being in this world can do, and that is to take conscious, corrective action. Animals act on instinct, or training. Human beings can experience things in a cognitive, aware state and take corrective action. If we get off course, we can bring ourselves back on course. We are blessed with that ability—when we use that ability.

1) Ask yourself, "What is my purpose in being here?" Answer out loud, or write down your answers, in a stream of consciousness way.

2) Choosing one of the answers you have said or written down, what small action can you take that would be in support of your purpose?

3) Keeping your eyes on your answer, and not letting yourself get distracted, hold with it until you move on some part of that action.

4) Continue this process every day until you feel yourself aligned and on course with your direction and purpose. *Note: It doesn't have to be* the *purpose of your life, but you will gain strength and healing from following any positive and loving course of action.*

5) Now attune to the essence of steadfastness inside you, and as an inner process, put it on or over the cause, indecision. You can also do this with a hand gesture, placing one palm on top of the other. Allow the cause of dis-ease to be transmuted into the cure of health and well-being. You can ask for the assistance of the Light in this process and remember to always ask for the highest good.

6) Describe how you are now feeling inside.

7) What have you learned?

# Cause
# 5

---

## INDIFFERENCE

Indifference may very well be the killer disease. Whether somebody hates you or loves you, they are involved with you. If I take my right hand and say that on the top of it there is love and on the underside of it there is hate, and if I start cutting away the hate, I'm going to end up with love. Even if I turn my hand the other way, it's still involvement. But when there's indifference, it's on the other hand, the left one. There is no love to get to. And there's no healing. It doesn't even care. You might as well be dead.

*Indifference is on the opposite side of love and hate.*

What most people want is to be recognized, loved, and appreciated. We can verbalize those by just saying, "I love you, I care about you. I want to know what you're doing, not out of meddling, out of caring for you. Because maybe I can assist you." That's called being a human being.

However, indifference kills the spirit inside. Indifference is on the opposite side of love and hate. And although the spirit can't really be killed, I'm trying to get across to you the serious impact indifference can have on your health and well-being. When we place negativity on our expression deep inside of us, called restraint, fear, restlessness, and indecision, the result is indifference.

1) Who comes to mind when you think of someone who has been indifferent to you?

2) Call in the Light and allow yourself to experience how you felt, or are feeling, about that.

3) Realize you can let it go by simply loving yourself and filling the emptiness.

4) Forgive yourself for judging that person or situation.

5) Is there someone or some situation that you are feeling indifferent towards right now? Describe how you feel inside.

6) Forgive yourself for judging yourself for shutting down any part of you.

7) Forgive yourself for judging the person or situation you feel indifferent towards.

# Cure

## 5

---

## GENTLENESS

What is the cure for indifference? Gentleness. The most powerful people on the planet are the most gentle because gentle people are strong, or they could not be gentle. Their egos are balanced, their thinking is balanced, they have a sureness about them, a natural confidence. They have been tried in the fires of negativity, and they have come out purified.

*The most powerful people on the planet are the most gentle because gentle people are strong, or they could not be gentle.*

It is like a very fine silver sword. The metal is dug up out of the ground and mixed with other elements, and then it is heated and pounded and put in cold water. This process is repeated over and over until the sword becomes very strong and refined. You must then hold this refined instrument very gently as it can cut with hardly any effort. That is the gentleness I am talking about.

Gentleness has a way to go in and cut out disease. Its main instrument is a kind word—not just a casual "please," but expressing loving appreciation from your heart and essence. When this appreciation comes from the heart in this gentle way, the other person knows it. This is important because most of the time we do not know how people feel about us. If you're not sure someone knows how much you appreciate them, tell them. They may not believe you, but that's theirs to sort out as you've told them the truth as you know it.

Should your husband or your wife, or anyone close to you, yell at you, just be thankful that they're involved with you. Instead of returning harsh words to match theirs, all you need do is cure them with gentleness. When they throw the hard ball of anger at you, you catch it and return the soft ball of gentleness. You play with it. Pretty soon their anger will be transformed into loving and upliftment.

1) Focus on your breath—its gentle rising and falling.

2) Start a process of infusing your body with gentleness. Begin by softening and relaxing your shoulders; and from there softening any areas of tension in your body.

3) Have this gentleness extend into your energy field around you.

4) Take a moment to stand or walk around in this gentleness.

5) Perceive this gentleness as a protective force field around you. Whatever enters this field is immediately softened and transformed into gentleness.

6) What kind words can you say to yourself?

7) What kind words can you say to someone close to you?

8) Now attune to the essence of gentleness inside you, and as an inner process, put it on or over the cause, indifference. You can also do this with a hand gesture, placing one palm on top of the other. Allow the cause of dis-ease to be transmuted into the cure of health and well-being. You can ask for the assistance of the Light in this process and remember to always ask for the highest good.

9) Describe how you are feeling inside.

10) What have you learned?

# Cause
## 6

___

### WEAKNESS

There is a weakness that I call the "tyranny of weakness." This is where someone plays that they are so very weak in order to have everybody running around doing things for them. These types of people are also very unhappy, because they never can rely upon themselves when troubles appear.

*And that weakness will be where your illness comes in and your disease lives.*

The tyranny of weakness is the power not to perform. It masquerades as "I'm not strong enough; it's too heavy for me to lift; I'll have to stay too long on my feet," and all sorts of other excuses. For example:

"I can't go. I have a headache." Get up and go.

"I can't water-ski. I don't know how." You won't learn sitting down. Get up on the skis.

"I'll fall." Yes.

"I can't swim." Put on a vest. Take a deep breath through it all.

"I can't sing." Practice.

"Oh, no. No!" Why not?

"Because I can't sing." I know, practice. Take lessons and get going.

"No. I'm protecting my weakness."

And that weakness will be where your illness comes in and your disease lives.

**Things to act upon and questions to ask yourself and ponder:**

1) Review your self-talk (this is what you say to yourself over and over again, day in and day out). What negative thing do you say to yourself consistently?

2) How can you turn that around to be positive?

3) Identify a pattern you have that you would regard as a weakness.

4) How are you protecting it?

5) What do you want to do but keep complaining that you can't do it?

6) How does that serve you in some way?

7) How can you turn that weakness into a strength?

8) Forgive yourself for any judgments that have surfaced.

# Cure
## 6

---

## STRENGTH

In every weakness there is a strength. A weakness of sickness has in it the strength to manipulate your spouse and others around you. When troubles and challenges come your way, that strength can be a blessing if you meet them head on.

*Strength is inner. Power is outer. I'm talking about inner strength.*

You meet the troubles and challenges through love, empathy, peace, steadfastness, and gentleness. Strength then follows automatically. It isn't hard work, like lifting weights; it's an inner strength. It's where you get goose bumps over your head as the spirit moves you. It's where you sit tall and strong inside. It's where you say, "Come what will, I'll handle it. I may not do it in the perfect way, but I'll handle it, and I'll grow from it." Not grow in it, grow from it. Don't grow in your disease; grow from your disease. There's a big difference. Some people grow in their disease, so they are very strong in fighting their disease, but they still have the disease. I'm talking about getting rid of it.

No matter what your illness is, get some strength in it because it needs it. Illness and strength are not compatible. One has to go. The strength will not go. Strength is inner. Power is outer. I'm talking about inner strength.

As I've said before, if you've made a mistake in your life, just call it a mistake and correct it. It's as simple as that. It's called owning it and taking authority over it. Taking authority over it produces strength.

1) When you think of a mistake you've made or a weakness you have, what comes to mind?

2) Mistakes and weaknesses can be portals to new awareness, so now see this mistake or weakness as a gift. What gift or blessing did you receive from this mistake or weakness?

3) As you own that gift and blessing, feel it strengthen you inside. What part of your body, mind, or emotions are feeling strengthened right now?

4) Experience your whole body being filled with an inner strength.

5) What are you aware of as this takes place?

6) Now get the essence of strength inside you, and as an inner process, put it on or over the cause, weakness. You can also do this with a hand gesture, placing one palm on top of the other. Allow the cause of dis-ease to be transmuted into the cure of health and well-being. You can ask for the assistance of the Light in this process and remember to always ask for the highest good.

7) Describe how you are feeling inside.

8) What have you learned?

# Cause

# 7

## DOUBT

Doubt is what I call having a double mind. Doubt says, "I want to do this, but what about this?" So there are now two things to do.

This type of doubt can be a burden and source of confusion. "I think so, but I doubt it." "I think I'm getting well, but I'm not sure." "I'm sure she loves me, but I don't know." "They might, but maybe they might not." It's often referred to as the evil eye because there is a lack of willingness to fully embrace the goodness in life. Someone may ask, "How's the day going for you?" and is answered, "It's just wonderful, except my back hurts."

When we are in a double mind, we are in a double bind and old doubts of years ago can come forward. In a marriage, when there is doubt in one person's mind, they may go into the past and bring up all their old grievances—even though at one time they were resolved. If that situation happens to you, you can say, "You must understand that fight is over; this is a new one. Fight fair."

I'll let you in on a secret—the brain isn't divided into right and left hemispheres. The brain is an associational organism.

1) What do you doubt about yourself?

2) What do you doubt about in others?

3) What do you doubt about the world?

4) You can prove your doubt, in which case it is no longer a doubt. If you can't prove your doubt, then let it go.

5) Observe how you second-guess yourself or hold back. What holds you back from fully embracing and owning your divinity?

6) Forgive yourself for any judgments you are holding against yourself or others.

# Cure
## 7

_____

## UNDERSTANDING

The cure for doubt is understanding even when there is no evidence to understand. You understand that doubt is part of the human condition, so you do not dwell upon your doubt but use it as a method to prove or disprove that which you're going towards. If you doubt something, go check it out. If it's not so, your doubt has been part of your knowledge. If it is so, your doubt has been part of your guidance system. Either way, you get to use doubt in a positive way.

*Let me remind you that everything that comes into your environment, internally or externally, you can use for your upliftment, learning, and growth.*

If you have love, empathy, peace, steadfastness, gentleness and strength—understanding appears. It is not an intellectual process. It comes out of the Spirit inside you. Through this understanding, you will be attuned to someone and know how they feel. If we truly knew the secret hurt of our worst enemy, we would never do one thing more to hurt them again. That's the truth. Think about that the next time you want to hurt somebody in any way, shape, or form. We all have our hurts.

If you have understanding, which is the cure for doubt, when doubt surfaces you can say, "I understand that I have doubt. That means there's something I don't know and that I am running assumptions about. I need more information."

Let me remind you that everything that comes into your environment, internally or externally, you can use for your upliftment, learning, and growth.

1) What if you did use everything for your upliftment, learning, and growth? How would the quality of your life change?

2) Understanding is a spiritual law. Right now, attune to the understanding that resides in your heart. What do you experience?

3) What does that understanding say to you?

4) Let go of any mental burdens you may be carrying, and move them into your heart where they can receive compassion and understanding.

5) Now get the essence of understanding inside you, and as an inner process, put it on or over the cause, doubt. You can also do this with a hand gesture, placing one hand on top of the other. Allow the cause of dis-ease to be transmuted into the cure of health and well-being. You can ask for the assistance of the Light in this process and remember to always ask for the highest good.

6) Describe how you are feeling inside.

7) What have you learned?

# Cause

## 8

---

### INTOLERANCE

Intolerance is a form of prejudice where you "know" something even before you know that you know. With intolerance, no matter what a person does, you can find something wrong with it. You make them wrong even if they're right.

Intolerance sounds like this: "Because you are not like me and you don't do it my way, you're wrong, and you're no good, so get out of here." It's also when you say, "I'm better than you, and I'm not going to listen to you." "I know it and you don't. Don't bother me."

**Things to act upon and questions to ask yourself and ponder:**

1) Whom, or what, do you make wrong? About what are you prejudiced?

2) When you think of this person or situation in (1) above, what do you feel in your body?

3) If you are aware that intolerance causes dis-ease in your body, take a moment to forgive yourself for any judgments you are holding against anybody or anything.

4) Fill the space where that intolerance resided with your loving.

# Cure

# 8

## TOLERANCE

The cure for intolerance is simple: it's tolerance, or patience. You can ask, "Tell me how you see it can be done in a better way." If you can be shown a better way, it's no longer intolerance; it's a correction. Then you accept the correction, do it better, and you lift yourself. So no matter what happens in your life, you use it to your advantage.

*We can't correct others' behavior, but we can certainly correct our own.*

Some people will be intolerant with you because you may be too tall, too short, male, female, blue eyes, brown eyes, wear glasses, no glasses, because you are from Colombia, the United States, Chile, or Germany. There's nothing you can do about those types of intolerance. It's not in your control, but it is in your control to be tolerant with the person next to you.

We can't correct others' behavior, but we can certainly correct our own. A person said to me once, "I don't like your suit." I said, "Wonderful, buy me a new one." Don't pick on anything unless you can correct it.

It is not the tolerance of procrastination that I am speaking about. It's the tolerance of finding out what someone is going through, what it is they are experiencing, and being present and patient with them.

1) Acceptance is the first law of Spirit. How accepting are you of yourself?

2) How accepting are you of others?

3) How accepting are you of the world?

4) Mock-up being unconditionally accepting, seeing everything as part of God's creation.

5) What effect does that have on your body, mind, and emotions?

6) How is your tolerance or patience inside you, right now?

7) Now get the essence of tolerance inside you, and as an inner process, put it on or over the cause, intolerance. You can also do this with a hand gesture, placing one hand on top of the other. Allow the cause of dis-ease to be transmuted into the cure of health and well-being. You can ask for the assistance of the Light in this process and remember to always ask for the highest good.

8) Describe how you are feeling inside.

9) What have you learned?

# Cause
# 9

---

## IGNORANCE

This is plain old ignorance. "How was I supposed to know? Nobody told me."

Did you think to ask? If you have a mouth, you could have.

When we don't hear something, we can have ignorance. But that ignorance can be corrected by listening. So ignorance is more than just not knowing; it's where we are not willing to know.

**Things to act upon and questions to ask yourself and ponder:**

1) What are you pretending not to know?

2) What are you ignoring about your body?

3) What are you not willing to see or acknowledge?

4) To whom do you give away your power?

5) What prevents you from asking more questions?

6) What are you scared of exploring?

7) Forgive yourself for any judgments that have surfaced.

.

# Cure

## 9

_____

# WISDOM

The cure for ignorance is wisdom. When you see someone studying, they are demonstrating wisdom, because that's how you learn the subject matter.

Someone once asked me, "How do I get more wisdom?" I answered, "In a word, practice! In two words, practice, practice. In three words, practice, practice, practice." I then said, "How many words do you need?" They said, "One, practice." That's how wisdom appears.

If you want to learn anything, practice. Practice makes it automatic, so then your intelligence can come forward also. So not only do you know how to spell a word, you also know how to put it in the sentence correctly. That's wisdom.

How do you get a lot of practice? Make a lot of mistakes. How do you make a lot of mistakes? Live your life in the fullest way you can with whatever situation you find yourself in and what you've got to deal with. Pretty soon you say, "Ah, I get it." That's also wisdom. It's also called insight.

*Live your life in the fullest way you can with whatever situation you find yourself in and what you've got to deal with.*

1) Take a moment to acknowledge the wisdom of your heart.

2) As you access that wisdom, what do you know to do that you are not doing in regard to your health and well-being?

3) What do you know not to do that you are doing in regard to your health and well-being?

4) What do you need to practice in relation to health and well-being?

5) How does your wisdom guide you into better health in this moment?

6) Now get the essence of wisdom inside you, and as an inner process, put it on or over the cause, ignorance. You can also do this with a hand gesture, placing one hand on top of the other. Allow the cause of dis-ease to be transmuted into the cure of health and well-being. You can ask for the assistance of the Light in this process and remember to always ask for the highest good.

7) Describe how you are feeling inside.

8) What have you learned?

# Cause
# 10

---

## IMPATIENCE

Maybe you are experiencing impatience now. "When is this book going to be over? I haven't read anything that I don't already know." Then why do you have health problems? It's because you know the information intellectually, as data, but you don't know it as the experience of living your life. That's the difference between information and experience. Information is of little use or value if you don't use it to bring forward the experience of transformation.

*Information is of little use or value if you don't use it to bring forward the experience of transformation.*

Impatience is hurry, hurry, hurry. "Hurry up! Get it to me, right now." Some things take time. Thinking takes time. However, to speak foolishly doesn't take any time at all. When people say to me, "Hurry," I say, "Do you want it to be good, or do you just want it?" If they want it to be good, then I tell them, "You must forgive me if I take a longer time to make it better for you." They inevitably say, "Take your time."

1) What pushes your buttons more than anything?

2) What are you impatient about?

3) Describe a situation in your life where you seem to be always in a hurry.

4) Describe something in your life that is not moving fast enough for you or that you want to be over?

5) What small (microscopic) step can you take towards improving your health?

6) If you had a timeline of a year to move towards a specific goal for greater health, and you were to make a microscopic step each day towards it, what would that goal be?

# Cure

## 10

---

## FORGIVENESS

The cure for impatience is forgiveness; not the forgiving of somebody but the forgiveness of your own impatience. You're demanding people to go too fast. So inside you, forgive yourself for demanding something they can't do.

*There's no real forgiveness until there is forgetting.*

If someone is judging you or berating you, and they are being impatient, maybe they don't have the necessary information. So you can ask them, "Show me how I can do it faster, the way you want it." Many bosses have turned around and walked away because they don't know how to do it faster either. They had the disease of impatience, and if they are smart, they can end up with the healing of forgiveness. In the state of forgiveness, they often find that they get what they want, and the quality of thankfulness soon follows.

Forgiveness has an emotional quality. But there's one a little higher, and that's called forgetting. When you've truly forgiven somebody, you forget it. Too many of us have said, "I've forgiven my mother and father for beating me almost to death when I was three years old." No, you haven't.

"Yes, I have forgiven them. I remember the stick they used."

Forget it.

"No, no way am I going to forget that."

There's no real forgiveness until there is forgetting.

1)  What is present for you to forgive?

2)  Forgive yourself for judging yourself, the person, or the situation.

3)  Forgive yourself for any hurt feelings or misunderstandings.

4)  Forgive yourself for the negative thoughts and images you have held in your mind.

5)  Forgive yourself for the negative fantasies that you have created around the situation.

6)  Allow your loving to fill the spaces where the negativity was.

7)  Allow God's unconditional loving, which is endless and infinite, to flood through you, washing away any sense of separation with yourself, people, the world, and your own divinity.

8)  Forgive yourself for forgetting that you are divine.

9)  Now get the essence of forgiveness inside you, and as an inner process, put it on or over the cause, impatience. You can also do this with a hand gesture, placing one hand on top of the other. Allow the cause of dis-ease to be transmuted into the cure of health and well-being. You can ask for the assistance of the Light in this process and remember to always ask for the highest good.

10) Describe how you are feeling inside.

11) What have you learned?

# Cause
# 11

## TERROR

Terror is fear of the unknown. Fear is when we think something is going to happen a certain way. Terror is of the unknown. But look at the funny thinking here: if it's unknown, why have terror, why not have ignorance? Why not have doubt, why not have anything but terror?

When a person has terror, they are trying to make you believe that they know what's going to happen. If they know what's going to happen, why are they standing there talking to you? They should get out of there. If you see somebody running fast, they may know what terror is. Don't stick around to find out what they are running from. Run with them and ask them, then you'll be as far along as they are!

Terror is also usually involved with the idea of "What if they leave me?" "What if they're taken away from me?" "Oh my god, what would I do?" Terror is a self-induced attachment to materiality with emotions running on top of it and a hallucination of what it might be. I have never found anything that could make me feel terror, except my own imagination.

**Things to act upon and questions to ask yourself and ponder:**

1) What situation or circumstance are you envisioning that elicits a sense of fear or terror in you?

2) What form of materiality are you attached to?

3) What comes to mind when you ask yourself the question, "Why am I attached to this form of materiality?"

4) What emotions surface when you think of losing this form of materiality?

5) What are you pretending to know that is, in actuality, unknown in this moment?

6) Forgive yourself for any judgments that have surfaced.

7) What can you shift inside to have more trust in God?

# Cure

# 11

## COURAGE

I cured my terror by using courage. The terror was in my own mind, so I walked up to what scared me and I looked at it completely. I was still scared, but there was no terror. But being scared was also an adventure. It's like a bull chasing you. When you don't stop to see if he's going to find you, it's exciting. If he finds you, that's terror!

*It takes courage, heart, to maintain the positive.*

Courage comes from a French word coeur meaning heart. Go to your heart and be loving. In that place of loving, terror does not exist. But courage can move out, and terror can move back in if you've set up a home for it. Some people are married to their negative patterns. They live in the negative more than the positive. Make sure you are not one of them. It takes courage, heart, to maintain the positive.

1) When you think of a courageous person, who comes to mind?

2) What do you admire about that person and what qualities do they demonstrate?

3) What if the qualities you are admiring are mirroring the qualities you have in you? Can you own them?

4) How can you demonstrate them?

5) What small step can you take today to activate and demonstrate courage?

6) What negative pattern do you repeat, habitually?

7) Are you willing to use and activate your courage and these other qualities to turn around negative direction into a positive direction?

8) Now get the essence of the courage inside you, and as an inner process, put it on or over the cause, terror. You can also do this with a hand gesture, placing one hand on top of the other. Allow the cause of dis-ease to be transmuted into the cure of health and well-being. You can ask for the assistance of the Light in this process and remember to always ask for the highest good.

9) Describe how you are feeling inside.

10) What have you learned?

# Cause
# 12

---

## GRIEF

When we have grief, it is because we are missing someone that we valued so much in this world. Maybe they died, or maybe they have a disease that they may die from. Maybe they are going away with somebody else or moving to another country. In these circumstances, grief is often something that says, "I cared too much." Often when we care more for a person than they care about us, an imbalance is created that can lead to grief.

*The feeling goes so deep that it can go into the very cells of your body.*

When you've lost somebody who has been really close to you, and you have invested a great deal of yourself in them, the depth of your grief cannot be told to somebody who has not had the experience. The feeling goes so deep that it can go into the very cells of your body.

**Things to act upon and questions to ask yourself and ponder:**

1) What are you grieving?

2) In which part of your body do you feel the grief?

3) Immerse that area of the body with loving.

4) See the cells in this area come alive with vibrant health.

5) Know that the Beloved holds you in Its arms.

6) Relax and let go into the Beloved.

# Cure

## 12

_____

## JOY

We can assist a person out of their grief by curing them with joy. Joy isn't something where you say, "Okay, let's have joy," although that can work. It's more about accessing enough joy inside so that it starts trickling out. Joy bubbles up and can make the body move and transform, and that's extremely important. Some people can't handle joy. It's too electrifying and can keep them awake. It's like a sugar rush.

*Joy bubbles up and can make the body move and transform, and that's extremely important.*

You may miss someone who has departed, but you also have the joy that you knew them and were able to spend time with them. I have great joy for what my parents taught me and that they were my parents. I miss them but have no grief, because they taught me what they knew. I would have grief if I didn't use what they gave to me, but I use it.

1) Joy, loving, and peace are qualities of the Soul. That means that these qualities are present in you, right now in this moment.

2) Forgive yourself for forgetting that you are divine.

3) Now attune to your divinity and go deeper inside you to where joy resides.

4) As you contact this vibration of joy, let it bubble up inside you, filling you to overflowing.

5) Visualize this joy moving through you and transforming and healing your body.

6) Allow yourself to smile inwardly (and perhaps outwardly).

7) Close your eyes and receive a blessing from Spirit, for your highest good.

8) Describe, or write down, the blessing you received.

9) Now get the essence of joy inside you, and as an inner process, put it on or over the cause, grief. You can also do this with a hand gesture, placing one hand on top of the other. Allow the cause of dis-ease to be transmuted into the cure of health and well-being. You can ask for the assistance of the Light in this process and remember to always ask for the highest good.

10) Describe how you are feeling inside.

11) What have you learned?

# Healing Through Spirit

## Light, Love, Sound, Breath

# Healing Light

**As you come present with yourself, allow the Light to flow through your body more and more, as you open to receive it. Relax every cell in your body to receive the Light.**

*John-Roger, D.S.S.*

*You are the Light. You are divine. You are in a state of becoming aware of what you already are.*

The Light is the energy of Spirit that pervades all levels of consciousness. It is an energy that is of God. It is pure, uncorrupted, and available for our use.

Spirit is energy, the force that activates the human consciousness and gives it life. Spirit individualizes itself as Soul and so resides closely within each consciousness. Many people have said that a human being has a Soul, but it is closer to reality to say that the Soul has a human being.

The Light is in everything; it's in every aspect of your experience and your expression. You have never been less than the Light. The Light is not sitting around, chanting, and looking holy all day. The Light is the total beingness of all consciousness, on all levels, at all times. The Light is everywhere. When you accept that, you've made your first step.

The presence of the Light is most active within the human consciousness, and the human consciousness is unique in its ability to be consciously aware of the Light and to work as a co-creator with the energy of Light.

There are two aspects of the energy of the Light. One is magnetic in nature, and you, consciously or unconsciously, are an individual director of it. When you work with this light for your highest good and for the highest good of everyone, you may also activate the spiritual Light. When you activate this higher Light (also called the Light of the Holy Spirit), you can experience at-one-ment with God.

This higher Light (the Holy Spirit) will never inflict itself on anyone or anything and comes only when invited. It can be active only when you are consciously pure in your intent and expression. You are pure in your expression when you ask for the Light to be present for the highest good. You do not condition the Light by asking it to do what you feel would be right or what you think would be right. When you just ask for the presence of the Light and ask Spirit to bring forward whatever is for the highest good, that is when you are L-I-G-H-T, that is, Living In God's Holy Thoughts.

*Wherever you go, ask for God's Light to surround you, protect you, and fill you for the highest good. Place it ahead of you wherever you are going so that you will always be well-received.*

The magnetic light is neither good nor bad; it depends on how it is used. It can be used, along with the spiritual Light, for those things that are positive and that enhance the spiritual evolution of each consciousness. The magnetic light can also be used in negative ways. Spiritual law says that all creations are returned to the creator, so it follows that any harm or hurt you perpetrate will be returned to you.

In the last few decades, a whole new consciousness has been moving across the planet. In that new consciousness, each person is found to be special, and as each develops their inner spiritual awareness, they have the ability to become attuned to the spiritual Light through their own consciousness. All people start their own salvation. I show you techniques, methods, and ways. I tell you what has worked for me and what I know has worked for other people, but it could all appear to be a lie until you do it and it works for you. This is why I always advise people to "check it out" for themselves and get their own experience.

Wherever you go, ask for God's Light to surround you, protect you, and fill you for the highest good. Place it ahead of you wherever you are going so that you will always be well-received. And each time you meet someone, ask that this Light be placed between the two of you, not as a barrier, but as that which can clarify. If you do that, everything that comes to you will come through the Light.

The Light works the way it works. It doesn't always work the way you think it should work or the way you would like it to work. It is the most powerful force on the planet and the most powerful force in your life. We use the expression "call in the Light," but the

Light is always here, so we actually call ourselves forward into the Light.

There are many techniques for asking for the Light, and the main idea is along these lines: "If this is for my highest good and for theirs, then I would like the Light to be placed with me, with them, and with this situation." If your intention is clear that you are asking for the spiritual Light for the highest good, you can also just say, "Light." This is the first thought in some people's minds when they hear a siren or hear about a situation that is distressing or challenging in some way. Some people read the newspaper and listen to news on TV, and in their consciousness is "Light" for all they read, hear, or see.

*Just ask for the Light to be there for the highest good. You aren't doing it; God is doing it. You are simply asking.*

There are a lot of ways to hold the Light and send the Light and work with the Light. One way is that as soon as someone tells you about a situation, just pass it right into the consciousness of the Light. Before that person even finishes getting the words out, the Light has gone.

Just ask for the Light to be there for the highest good. You aren't doing it; God is doing it. You are simply asking. If all things are happening according to the highest good and in perfect timing, why send the Light? Because Spirit will not usually look at a plan to see if an alternate can be instituted unless requested from this level of Spirit.

On this level where most of us function, all things don't necessarily happen for the highest good or in perfect timing. So it's always appropriate to send the Light for the highest good (which is something God knows and we, in our personality levels, don't always know). Sending the Light for the highest good increases the positive energy in a situation and increases the likelihood that the highest good possible will take place, rather than a not-so-high good.

Keep it simple. Sending the Light does not have to be complicated. You don't have to spell out all the details. All you need to do is place the situation in God's hands and let God handle the results.

Thoughts are transmitted over long distances, and they can affect us on many different levels. This is why just sending the simple thought of "I love you" or "God bless you" can work wonders. If someone you know is having difficulties with their health, when you meditate, see them healthy, whole, and balanced. Hold that positive image. Send them the Light, for the highest good, and keep your emotions neutral. As you maintain loving, positive energy flowing out to them, it can be of great support and, as they allow it through their openness, it will assist them in their recovery.

*When you receive a Spiritual healing, there is one thing that follows: a necessity of change.*

The Light works through medical doctors, chiropractors, osteopaths, acupuncturists, massage therapists, and many others. Some of them heal with this Light much more often than they heal with any other factor. Why? Because medicines and other interventions do one of two things, they either stimulate or depress. They stimulate the body so it will get going or they depress the body so it won't over-create. Everything else is done inside your body.

When you receive a Spiritual healing, there is one thing that follows: a necessity of change. You cannot receive a healing from cancer and go on wishing to die. You will wish the cancer back into your system. You can't go along being healthy and envisioning yourself in a car wreck. You must change that thing within your creative consciousness that is producing this thrust into the negative.

Principle #6 on page 49 states, "Create a system of self-talking that talks you into greater vitality and health." If you are being a responsible creator, you can say, "Father, I really don't know what's going on, and I'm open to suggestion. I ask that the Christ consciousness be with me to help me get through this dis-ease that I am manifesting, and if it can be resolved into the Light and not through my body, then I choose that."

I would also say, every day, "Divine love floods my consciousness with health and every cell of my body is filled with Light."

# Healing Light Meditation

## 1

---

If you are open to it, we are going to work with a healing Light, here and now. Just follow along and do your best to envision what I am saying as you read the words. Always ask for "the highest good of all concerned" when you work with the Light.

See a bright Light being placed in the center of your forehead. This Light stretches upward and outward (to the sides and backwards and forwards), like a three-dimensional cross. Now see this going around the head, in a band, and also circling around the top of the head and down through the neck and back around to the chin.

Now you move the Light from the forehead down into the throat area. This Light is an amber color and it is beautiful. It's circling around your neck. This can help a sore throat or a kinked neck that you may have woken up with this morning.

Now see this Light moving down to your heart. It actually seems to be percolating the blood. The blood is being purified with this action; it's being filtered.

Now this Light starts to have a thicker or heavier quality, so you can be more aware of its presence as it surrounds you.

Keep your hands separated as the Light now moves from your heart right into the palms of your hands. You'll probably start feeling it more directly here, this presence of this Holy Spiritual Light, as it manifests for you, working in those areas that are in need of healing and balance.

Now feel a great peace descending on you with this Light. As you tune your body more to this high vibratory rate, you feel it starting to go up and down your spine, bringing your posture into alignment. You find yourself naturally sitting up straight when that Light goes up and down your spine.

It even goes down into the lower buttocks area where the Kundalini force resides. This Light is stirring and loosening and bringing balance. This area can be a source of confusion and so just relax as the Light activates and charges this center to align its duties. For women having problems in this lower area, it might feel like a hot needle or hot match being touched in there.

This Light is now moving around your body. It may be working on your knee or your throat. Just accept and receive and flow with this Light's vibratory rate. For God's will is being done.

Now take in, through your nostrils, a deep breath and hold it for a moment. And let it out. Breathe in again, hold it, now release it. One more time, breathe in, hold it, and let it out. Now relax as this Light just keeps circling the body.

Don't try to make anything happen. Most of us try way too hard. Let it touch to you. Once again, ask for the Light of the Christ and the Light of the Holy Spirit to surround, protect, and fill you at this time.

Take this amber Light now and place it in the middle of the room. Within this Light, send a mental image of your loved one to whom you'd like to send the spiritual healing.

Now place within that Light those who you feel have not been your friends. And ask for this Light to bless them.

Take your left hand and bring it up in front of you like you'd be saying "halt" to someone. "Halt" is facing outward. Can you feel the presence of the Light? Place the right hand upward in your lap. Don't lift it, just turn it up.

Now raise your right hand up about half way and turn it outwardly like you are blessing someone. Have your right hand a little lower than your left. You should be able to feel the difference in those hands.

Without touching them together, turn both hands to face you. Bring them up towards your face very slowly, until you can feel the energy of your hands on your face. Again, don't touch yourself.

Now take your hands around to your ears, and bring them just a little closer in and feel the wave of Light as it goes in your ears. It may sound something like a roaring ocean. You may also feel it as a pulsating energy, perhaps feeling this pulsating a little more in one hand than the other.

Very slowly bring your hands down in your lap like you're holding a baby. And just hold yourself in a relaxed position until you feel the Light lift away from you.

As you learn how to increase your Light and increase the frequencies of your body and consciousness, you are then able to give this Light to other people. I call it Light Ability. It can be conveyed silently, by the spoken word, the written word, or by touch. Many times it's conveyed by our changing our own behavior and habits into a higher frequency. One way you can tell whether someone is a Light worker is that there is Light in their eyes.

# Healing Light Meditation

## 2

_____

Here is another healing Light attunement:

*Just envision the healing Light of God going all through your body. As you feel this, you may also feel your body frequency being lifted.*

Now as we tune in to that oneness that is the Spirit, we ask for quietness within our Souls and our minds and our bodies. Father Mother God, we ask now to be placed within the Light of the Christ allowing only that which is for our highest good to be brought forward. We would ask for this now in perfect love and perfect understanding, keeping in mind our destinies on this planet. We are glad to be of service again, Father, and for this we always give our thanks. Thy will be done.

You feel this holy Light descending on you now. It's starting to come down like a blanket. Have your legs uncrossed and your hands separated with your palms facing upward and just relax. Receive in a deep breath, and as you exhale, let go of any negativity. You don't "try" to do anything in this attunement; you just relax and let the Spirit touch to you.

Just envision the healing Light of God going all through your body. As you feel this, you may also feel your body frequency being lifted. A green healing Light now starts to appear, and as it does, be open to the possibility of a healing taking place within you. Perhaps if you have had stiffness in your neck, see this green healing Light on it. If you've been tight and tense in the stomach area, see the green healing Light coming into that area. If you've been experiencing doubt, the Light is in on that doubt, so just relax and receive it as it comes in right now.

Now this Light continues to work with you as you receive it in the silent worship of your own Soul. This is your chance to move into higher consciousness right now. Feel yourself lifting up. Let your heart soar upwards. Let your mind soar upwards. Let all things fall away from you except you and the Presence of God. Let the presence of this immense peace and calm come into you.

Whatever you need right now for your spiritual growth, just see it in this Light bringing it to you, for your highest good. If you need healing for a part of your body, whichever part needs Light, just see that part perfect inside you. There's nothing impossible with Spirit, because everything is from Spirit.

The Light lifts that consciousness, and it can detoxify, cleanse, purify, and heal. You have this spiritual healing Light working with you now. Just accept as it comes into you, in this moment.

*The Light lifts that consciousness, and it can detoxify, cleanse, purify, and heal.*

You can say a prayer right now: "Father, I receive. I accept all things. My joy in your Presence lifts me higher. Father I worship you. I move forward in my Light consciousness. I accept my divinity and know that where God is, nothing else can be other than in a perfect state."

Now send the Light to those in need. You see these people being placed in the Light. If you prefer, you can even say their names out loud or silently within you, and you let the Light go to them for their highest good. Their highest good may be that the Light not reach them because of what's going on in their lives, but this Light will circle around them and wait until they ask God for help. It will move in and bless them with its presence.

Even if you have had disturbances with people, place them now in this Light and remember to place yourself there also and receive. You receive through the opening of your consciousness. If you give a little, you receive a little. It is your choice, but you should know what the choices are.

Just relax until you feel the Light lift away. And know that you can call yourself forward into it at any time.

As a reminder, Light is Living In God's Holy Thoughts, and each person does it according to his level of consciousness and according to each level of being the Light. This type of Light is the invisible Light, the healing Light, the all knowing Light. You and I are Light. Everyone of us is Light.

Some of you have got your bulbs turned on inside, while others are still trying to find out where you plug it in. Some of you are trying to exchange your bulb for a higher wattage, so that you can go on with your lives in a higher frequency. Each person has to do it in their own unique way, but you're never alone when you tune into divine love.

The love of looking at a newborn baby is divine love. The look of two young lovers is divine love. It is all divine love when we have placed the highest good of that person ahead of our actions towards them. You know it's very hard to love in a divine way because it can't be understood with the mind. It's spiritual. This oneness with all humanity is within the heart of every being.

Many people reading this book will receive divine love until their cup runs over. Many others will receive just a little cupful. But even a little bit is a fantastic amount.

# Healing Love

Since loving is the keynote of my work in Soul transcendence, I have spoken a lot about it in this book *(see Principle #8, page 61, and Stages of Healing #7, page 204)*. Here are a few more words on the subject that will hopefully inspire you to go to the source of healing within you.

Let's start by having you visualize the very best of yourself—the joy and the loving flowing within you and out of you—and hold that vision inside you. As you hold that vision, it will become a reality because that's the real you. Essentially, I'm asking that you go to the place that responds when you hold a child, the place that awakens when you help someone just for the pleasure of doing it. Connect with the sacred energy that comes alive when you express loving.

*Love is the healer. Joy is the expression.*

Long ago, I told myself that whenever a feeling of depression came over me, it would immediately move me to joy. In other words, I reprogrammed depression for happiness. Anything less than a state of loving can be used to reprogram you back into a state of loving. Anything off-center can be used to move you back to center.

Joyfulness and loving—love in action—are expressions of the true self. This form of loving is not to be confused with romantic love. Romantic love is conditional: we love someone for what they will do for us or give us, and once they stop giving us what we want, we withdraw our love and give it to someone else we think will fill our needs. The loving expression of the true self is giving, free, and unconditional.

When loving is unconditional, it is not dependent on how others behave. We continue to love someone regardless of what they do or say. We may not condone their behavior, and we may choose not to be with them, but our love for them is not conditioned in any way. Unconditional love is like that of a mother for her child. No matter what the child does—poops, cries, poops again

—the mother's loving remains a constant, consistent, and nonjudgmental presence.

So don't let anything you do—no matter how wrong or petty or shameful it seems—stand in the way of your loving. Let your loving embrace every part of you, because that loving, and the joyfulness that comes with it, is truly who you are. Practicing joy and loving is more fun than practicing depression, anxiety, and fear. Put yourself in training for Soul consciousness by practicing the positive aspects of living and loving.

*Above all, practice being loyal to your Soul. You do that by loving yourself through all your experiences and realizing that there is no value in putting yourself down. There are far better choices to make, and the best one is to love it all.*

Whenever you find that you are out of touch with your loving, simply move into the quiet center within. Let go of any expectation that something has to happen. When you are free of any pressure to perform that you have placed on yourself, and you become still, love arises naturally. Sometimes it's when you do nothing that the loving appears in its clearest form.

In our outer lives our satisfaction often depends on circumstances. But the inner life of loving, joy, and relaxation is fulfilling regardless of circumstances. If you can take just one day and live it with full awareness that you are completely responsible for whatever happens, and if you can observe yourself neutrally and lovingly in the process, you will be transformed. You will see everything as perfect and will realize that life really is as simple as breathing in and breathing out.

Above all, practice being loyal to your Soul. You do that by loving yourself through all your experiences and realizing that there is no value in putting yourself down. There are far better choices to make, and the best one is to love it all. One way you can learn to maintain the Soul center, which is oneness with God, is to bring together all aspects of your life's expression in the attitude of loving.

You cannot control circumstances from the outside. So instead of resisting pain and failure and defending against it, you can embrace and encompass your pain and your failures, fully accepting them so that they become part of you. You then can let them go because they are part of your inner environment—they are within your domain—and the loving of your Soul can dissolve them.

You can deal with any challenge in this way: lovingly extend your energy field and encompass the situation, then maintain a sense of neutral observation. This approach places you securely in your center, the Soul. Then, from this center, spiritual energy starts radiating outward. It does not radiate out as personality, but as an expression of your Soul's Light.

If you will strive to have a pleasant disposition while you're doing whatever you're doing in the world, there is a greater tendency for your Soul, which is so perfect and so loving, to radiate out of your pleasant disposition. A truly pleasant disposition is loving, compassionate, and empathetic, with the ability to know what's going on in the world, because it is not run by the ego. If you take that same pleasantness back inside you, you live with an abundance of enthusiasm that overflows to others. Now that is truly helping the planet.

*When the loving heart is flowing and functioning, it has no wants and desires—none.*

When the loving heart is flowing and functioning, it has no wants and desires—none. It is the emotions that want this and that. When you're neutral and unattached, you don't care what anyone else does. But you care that you're loving and open and that you're expanding your consciousness. What if it doesn't expand at the rate you want? You're not neutral as soon as you entertain that thought. You're intellectualizing and may be setting a trap for yourself. Instead of listening to the intellect, listen to your heart.

You practice being in the presence of Soul by being flexible and open in your mind and emotions, by looking at people and loving the good and the bad equally. Should you love others more than you love yourself? No, because it is through loving yourself unconditionally that you enter into the Spirit that resides within you. That's when you become a real joy to be around. That's when you discover the Soul.

The loving that is the true self's nature comes with sharing and caring. No matter how loving you feel, if you do not share your love, then you will simply be feeding your ego. But if you are caring and sharing, your loving opens the personality. Then the exterior senses can be utilized by the Soul, so that we naturally see where best to invest our efforts for the greater good of all.

Loving unconditionally does not mean that you have to participate with someone in their actions. That is their expression and their opportunity to learn, not necessarily yours. Loving unconditionally means that you accept their action without judgment and without being emotionally reactive.

There is one positive thing we can do with our thoughts; we can use them to keep remembering who we are—loving beings. It's so easy to get caught up in the stress of life today and forget that. We rarely stay focused on an idea for three seconds before our attention spins off into other thoughts, often negative ones of depression, anxiety, rejection, and fear. Then the body tenses up.

Wouldn't it be nice if our bodies were relaxed and peaceful, our emotions joyful, and mentally we were free? Freedom isn't the license to do what you want, it's the ability to be who and what you are—until you realize that you are the sky and that you are connected with and part of the very essence of all things. Then you don't have to play the game of separation, lack, or unworthiness. You open to the essence of who you are, which is much greater than any thought or feeling. And you awaken to the knowledge that the spiritual sky is all of us.

When you were a baby learning to walk, you didn't scold yourself when you fell down. You got up and tried again. Falling is just part of the process of learning to walk. This is the model for how we learn anything, including how to live. It's all about bringing ourselves back to the present, again and again. We love, then forget to be loving, then remember, and become loving again. The more we remember to love, the more habitual loving will become. It's a matter of being present in every moment.

You are never outside of God, whatever you do, but if you express yourself negatively, you may separate yourself from your awareness of God. Express loving in all ways, always, and you will know the presence of God in your life.

# Healing Sound

**Best of all is to preserve everything in a pure, still heart, and let there be for every pulse a thanksgiving, and for every breath a song.**

*Konrad von Gesner*

You can perceive your very breathing process as a form of patience. What would happen if you tried to take all the rest of your breaths right now? You'd probably explode. It would be too much to handle. So you take them one after another, in their proper timing. You let your breathing take care of itself, knowing that it is set up to do just that. And, without any effort, you're pretty patient towards that process. For the most part, the breaths are taken gradually. You can speed them up, but then you get the results of that too, which might be too much energy and a little hyperventilation. So you then slow the breathing down to bring it into a balance, into a harmonious rhythm.

In every season, there is a rhythm, and in every person, there is a rhythm. This rhythm has an innate intelligence that naturally moves and flows with what is going on. When you can tune into your inner rhythm (maybe for you it's a concerto, a waltz, or a march), you can sense its flow and relax into it. You then live a divine melody.

As you sit and listen to your rhythm within, you can amplify it and build on it to create the beautiful symphony that truly represents the divine spark of God within you. But it needs to be done gradually within the rhythm that is very particularly yours.

The sound inside you is the Sound of God. But sometimes, when you are distracted by the difficulties in your world, you won't pause long enough to listen to the sound and the assistance coming from within you. When you have a difficulty or feel stuck, you can start the attunement to Spirit by chanting "HU" (pronounced

*As you chant the healing tones, they create a higher vibration rate inside you. You keep going until the sound starts to fill the entire physical body. As it does that, it starts to clean and clear the body and raise the vibration of the cell level itself. It's a purification process that dissolves anger, anxiety, and other negative emotions.*

like hue) or "ANI-HU" (pronounced ahn-eye hue). (More detailed information on the HU and ANI-HU follows in this chapter.)

We can approach the chanting of these healing sounds by bringing them to life with our breath and our intent, just like a musician brings music to life through the playing of an instrument. We begin in silence and let our breath initiate the sound from within us. We then return to silence and appreciate its deeper, more refined quality. We can again, through the breath, enter into communion with God or Spirit and then repeat the sound or maintain the inner silence.

When chanting inwardly or out loud, relax your shoulders and your jaw and let the sound flow through you like a wave. Enjoy the quality of relaxation and healing it brings. Just be open and experience the sacredness and feel how God is embracing you and loving you. Then add your own quality of loving—loving every part of yourself—and feel the wave-like movement of the sound going through you, being amplified by the Beloved. Allow this sacredness to fill the temple that is your body, and as it vibrates with love and Light and sound from the chanting, you once again return to the silence.

## Healing Sound: THO

The THO Meditation is a marvelous but underutilized resource that we have for healing.

The word "THO" is a very powerful word that can be used as a mantra to bring healing to the body. It has been used since ancient times by the masters of the mystery schools to bring in a healing vibration. When you intone the word in the correct way, you pull to yourself a healing vibratory rate. It increases the energy that is within you and brings a flowing power into the consciousness.

This word is a sacred word, as are all the tones taught in this chapter. They are not to be taken lightly or used for purposes other than the upliftment of the consciousness.

As with the other meditations, you begin this one by coming into a state of quiet, asking the Light to surround, protect, and fill your consciousness, and asking that the meditation bring to you that which is for your highest good.

To bring forward the healing frequency, the tone must be said a certain way. It's almost the same idea as a voice graph. If the right person—one who knows the "key"—says the right word, he can open the vault. The same word said incorrectly will have no effect. The tone of THO said incorrectly will have no effect. Said correctly, it is extremely powerful.

The mantra, the tone, is combined with a pattern of breath control. Both the tone and the breath control are equally important to the whole effect.

1. Breathe in deeply and hold the breath—then exhale fully.

2. Breathe in again, hold it—and exhale fully.

3. Breathe in deeply, for the third time, and this time then exhale forcefully, sharply, saying aloud, "THoooo." The emphasis is on the "TH" sound, with the "ooooh" sound trailing for a second or two.

   The "TH" is a sharp, percussive sound. The "ooooh" sound is held for a second or two, and then all the rest of the air is exhaled.

4. Breathe normally for a minute or so and then repeat — three deep breaths, holding the air in for a few seconds and then exhaling fully, saying the tone "THoooo" on the third exhalation.

5. Breathe normally for a minute and then repeat once more.

We don't suggest you repeat the mantra more than three times in any one session. If you're doing it correctly, you will feel a tremendous power build up just in three repetitions. After you have done this aloud for some time, you may want to try it silently. It will carry great power done silently, too; but to learn it and attune yourself to it, it's best done out loud.

You may find that the mantra is most effective when you breathe in through your nose and out through your mouth—and the exhalation on the first two breaths should take approximately twice as long as the inhalation.

When you have finished the mantra, close your eyes, rest quietly, and observe the inward action. Since this is a mantra of healing, you may very well see the color green. This is the primary color that will come forward. You may also see some gold or blue with the green. In some cases, the green blends with the blue and the color will look turquoise. It will often come in swirling patterns, creating funny shapes and swirls of energy.

This mantra will bring in the healing power, and it will be condensed primarily around the head area first. So you may feel this as pressure, pulsating, or lightheadedness. Let that all be okay. Then as you sit quietly and let the power work, it will come down through the body and concentrate on those areas that are in need of healing.

It works through all levels of the consciousness to bring it all into balance. But if you wish, you can direct it into those areas that you feel are out of balance by just focusing your attention onto the areas in need of balancing and seeing them healthy and perfect. (Don't direct this energy to the eyes. The energy is already concentrated in that area, and an extra "dose" can make the eyes go out of focus and make you dizzy.)

As you sit in quiet meditation after intoning "THO," you can just picture other people in your creative imagination, and this healing power will go to them, also.

This mantra is a powerful force. It alters the energy patterns around the body. It changes them. If you find yourself in tense situations at work, for example, you might want to do this tone inwardly, and it may very well start altering the energies around you. Things may start becoming calmer and more balanced. But remember that you never, ever use these sacred tones of God to force a control pattern on anyone. Use them for your own balance and your own upliftment, and if that brings balance and upliftment to others, then that's great.

If you use these tones to control, then you have entered into black magic and brought karma to yourself. You will be held responsible for your actions. Do yourself a favor and don't enter into that area. Just work with these tones to bring yourself into greater health and balance, to expand and lift your consciousness, and to assist you on your path of upward evolution towards God realization.

## Healing Sound: HU

The "HU" tone reflects an ancient name of the Supreme God, and it invokes the purity of that perfect God. It may be chanted several ways. One way is to separate it into its letters "H" and "U" and chant it that way.

If you are chanting it out loud, you may take in a deep breath and then, as you breathe out, chant, "H..." "U..."

If you are chanting silently, you might intone the "H..." as you breathe in, and the "U..." as you breathe out.

You can also pronounce the "HU" as one syllable (pronounced "hugh") and chant it as you breathe out.

A very effective way to work with this HU chant is to do some deep breathing before you begin the chant. Breathe in and out five times, feeling the body filling up more and more with the Light energy on each breath, bringing yourself into calm, into your center, as you breathe.

After five breaths, begin the chant by breathing in and chanting the "HU" as you exhale. Do this for five breaths. Then repeat the process: five breaths without the chant and five with the chant. Then repeat it one more time—so that you chant the "HU" fifteen times in all. This will build up terrific energy. Once you have done this series of fifteen, I would suggest waiting at least fifteen minutes before you try it again—and you probably won't want to do that more than twice each day.

This tone can be chanted silently, as an ongoing chant, at almost any time and place. It can really be helpful in centering yourself and bringing balance to yourself.

The HU can open your spiritual consciousness, thus bringing awareness to other levels. Because of this, I strongly recommend that you do not chant it while you're driving or operating machinery.

## Healing Sound: ANI-HU

The "ANI-HU" chant is a variation of the "HU" chant. This is chanted as you breathe out if you are chanting out loud. If you are chanting silently, you might chant the "ANI" as you breathe in and the "HU" as you breathe out—or the entire tone as you breathe out. Do whatever feels most comfortable to you. You may find yourself doing it one way one day and the other way the next day. These tones are given to you, and it's flexible how you work with them. You work with them in the way that they will work best for you. Don't be afraid to experiment.

The "ANI-HU" chant is also an invocation to the pure one, the Supreme God, but it has an added dimension that brings in the quality of empathy with others. As you chant this tone, you will find that quality of empathy increased. For this reason, it is a beautiful chant to do in a group situation as a continuous, rolling sound. In a large group, it can begin to sound like "And I, You" or "You and I" …"ANI-HU-ANI-HU-ANI…

## Healing Sound: HOO

The "HOO" (pronounced WHO) chant is a very similar frequency to the "HU." Some people will feel more of an attunement with one, some with the other. They may be used interchangeably.

The "HOO" is chanted as a one-syllable tone and, if used in a group, as a continuous, rolling tone. As the focus and concentration is placed in the center of the head while chanting, the scattered energies of the body (sexual, physical, emotional, and mental) will be lifted and brought together in greater balance. This tone frequency is slightly lower than the "HU" or "ANI-HU."

## Healing Sound: WH-HOO

This is a variation of the HOO. The WH (pronounced like the "wh" in white) adds a very effective healing frequency to the tone. It can be chanted inwardly or out loud, in a group or alone.

Once again, always call the Light of the Holy Spirit for the highest good of all concerned to be present with you and around you. Then feel free to experiment with how this tone can work best for you. For example, you can experiment with chanting it inwardly on the inhale or out loud on the exhale. You can bring the tone through your whole body or, alternatively, isolate a part of your body you wish to bring care and attention to.

# Healing Breath

Student, tell me, what is God?
He is the breath inside the breath.

*Kabir*

God breathes through us so completely…
so gently we hardly feel it… yet it is our everything.

*John Coltrane*

When you breathe in, Spirit comes into you. That's why it is often valuable to begin spiritual exercises by focusing on your breathing. Bring the breathing under conscious control for a little while. Breathe deeply. Envision the Light of Spirit and of God coming into your body with each breath. Take the time to consciously move your breath—and, with it, the Spirit—through your body. This can bring great relaxation, renewal, and healing.

There is something about your next breath. That next breath is how close you are to Spirit. That's your source of energy right there in front of you. That's the Spirit, the energy, the Light, all of it, right there. Take that next breath as if you really were—and you really are—breathing in the essence of Spirit. Use that Spirit and that energy to sustain you in your life pattern. Use it to lift into the true self that you know is really you and into the consciousness of your own Soul and the awareness of the supreme God.

Your breath is one of your greatest allies. It is the key to restoring your energy. It is mentioned a lot in this book, but here are some keys and reminders:

Just the simple act of following the rising and falling of your breath can bring you to a peaceful and calm place and restore your energy. It also brings you into the ever-present, but often elusive, now.

Allowing the breath into the belly is one of the best things you can do to reduce stress.

The key to natural and full breathing is in the exhalation—the letting go. However, don't force anything. As you observe the exhale, you may be aware of a slight pause. This is natural, just observe. Then, without forcing anything, open to receive the next breath into you.

Place the breath anywhere in your body where you have tension, anywhere it feels lifeless or numb. You may find that as you bring the breath into that part of your body, what felt "dead" starts to come "alive."

To find harmony, you can always begin by getting out of the past. There is absolutely no need to think about yesterday or last week. Just tell yourself to stop doing that. Don't waste time thinking about tomorrow; forget it. Do nothing except—right now—feel where your body is, feel your feet on the ground. Take in a deep breath. Enjoy that breath and as you let it out, release the strain from yourself. Receive of the next breath and let it go. All that is necessary right now is to follow your breathing. You are present with yourself in the most simple, unadorned, and complete way.

Leave the memories to others and come present in the reality of this breath. Many teachers say that a good technique for overcoming difficulties is to concentrate on your breathing and watch yourself breathe. That can be difficult to do, because breathing is such a habitual response that you forget to focus on it consciously. While you're watching your breathing, you start thinking, "I wonder if anybody else is watching their breathing? They're probably out playing golf." And instantly, you're with them playing golf in your mind and forget that you're supposed to be watching your breathing.

If you find that you are hurrying, pressuring yourself, if you have a preoccupation or worry that is robbing you of energy, or you notice that your shoulders are a little high and tense, pause. Take a breath—rest in the moment and slowly allow your shoulders to lower, and your emotions to let go.

A further refinement is to bring your attention to the pause between exhaling and inhaling. Even doing this once will give you a moment of rest and restoration. All you really and truly have to do is continue breathing. For the truth is that with each breath you take, God is saying to you, "I'm right here. Everything is fine." That is the eternal essence of God that is entirely present at every moment.

Your next breath is your most important breath. Take it. If you didn't, you wouldn't be here. That's really living now. Each breath lifts you to a new level. From that new level, as you watch your next breath, you can slip away from everything extraneous to you. Then it becomes so joyful to take that next breath. You realize that the breath keeps the body going so that the Soul can reside in this temple and express on this level to all other manifestations of the Beloved.

Breathe in divine energy, let it work through you, and then let it go. Just as you let your next breath go, so you can let go of your wants, cravings, desires, and tension. As much as you can imagine God, you miss it. As much as you can feel God, you miss it. And as much as you can think about God, you miss it. But as soon as you turn into your own breath, and beyond to that which activates your breath, you can once again experience God. You can live without food for a long period of time, and you can live without water for a while. But you die without your next breath, and the next breath is the Spirit.

The Spirit comes in on your breath. It is that close—or closer. Even if you would try to deny the Spirit by holding your breath, the Beloved is that which will be there when your consciousness passes out from lack of oxygen. It will function behind the consciousness and keep the breath going anyway. It will allow you to pass out, restore the breathing, and awaken you.

There are many techniques to breathing that can be found in most Yoga books. For our purposes in this book, we want to focus on breathing that creates calm, relaxation, and well-being.

Moving the belly with the breath, also known as diaphragmatic breathing, triggers the parasympathetic nervous system and induces calm. Dr. Bruce McEwen calls it the single most important thing we can do to reduce stress.

During times of high stress, it's common to tense the upper chest and tighten the muscles in the shoulders and throat. When we're at rest, the muscles of the upper chest are soft and relaxed as we breathe, and the lower rib cage is more engaged. Consciously relax the jaw, throat, neck, and shoulders, and envision the breath flowing in and out of the deepest parts of the lungs as you breathe in and out.

Relaxation is a huge key. When we are relaxed and at ease, our exhalations become longer than our inhalations. In fact, an excellent way to get into a more relaxed state is to extend the length of our exhalations. Under stress our exhalations can be short and choppy, but when we relax they become fuller and longer.

The relaxed state also assists with our achieving a short pause after the exhalation. This pause is a brief but refreshing way to gently rejuvenate. It can be a sacred moment of stillness in a busy day.

The ancient Chinese sage Chung-Tzu advised, "Breathe into your heels." Breathe with and through your whole body. A sleeping baby is a perfect example of this. Let your breath bathe every cell with oxygen, love, and light. When we're relaxed, the alternating rhythm of the inhalations and exhalations feels like a gentle wave—soft, smooth, and uninterrupted. Consciously relaxing into this wave-like, oceanic quality of the breath deepens our sense of peace and ease.

Can you observe how each breath is radiating vitality all through your body to even the minutest part—to every system, organ, tissue, and cell? The more you relax with your breathing, the more you're conscious of the one breath in all things. More and more you experience your breath reaching to God until you breathe with God. And God breathes you with the love of the Divine.

# The Stages of Healing

In this section, you can take the key area of health imbalance that you are working on or looking to improve and put it through the healing stages.

Always ask for the Light for the highest good before beginning the process.

# Healing Stage
## 1

---

## PEACE

Peace is the absence of againstness. It is where there is no war within yourself or with others. You can take both sides of any point of view and look at them neutrally and with discernment, with no need for getting agitated, upset, worrying, or carrying on a negative conversation in your mind.

*This is the peace of you living your life and doing your work without any terror, fear, or negative fantasizing. For once you have established peace within your own consciousness, no one can take it from you.*

This is an inner peace. It's not sitting in a corner saying, "I'm having peace." That's stale, stagnant, and sitting in a corner. This is the peace of you living your life and doing your work without any terror, fear, or negative fantasizing. For once you have established peace within your own consciousness, no one can take it from you. They won't even be able to find it, and they certainly won't be able to dislodge it.

It's very simple to know when you are expressing peace. If you accept someone who is different, peace is present. If you move past your emotions and judgments into understanding and empathy, peace is being expressed. If you are being loving, peace reigns.

As you breathe in peace, tensions and worries drop away, and peace starts radiating through your body. Peace is present. As you drop the pressures of your life, you'll find that peace is very much alive and present, beyond all the distractions of the world.

You can practice using what I call the nine magic words. The first three are "I love you." The second three are "God bless you." And the third three are "Peace, be still."

Say them silently when you are in situations of conflict or upset. These words are powerful. They bring peace.

Make peace with yourself. Forgive yourself for all the times you haven't done your best, no matter what the reason. Forgive yourself for forgetting that you are divine.

Peace is not holding a position about anything or anyone, and you do not judge. Peace is neutrality, where you are not for or against anything or anyone. You are in a middle ground of acceptance, which frees you up for positive, loving action.

To move into a situation or towards a goal peacefully means that you are bringing peace and harmony into what you are doing. The opportunity to be in peace is in every moment, in every choice. You come into peace first with yourself and then you share peace with others.

You are your own health machine. You are your own destruction machine. Let your motto be: "Let there be peace on earth, and let it begin with me."

## Applying the Stages of Healing: PEACE

1. Realize that peace is present inside of you, right now.

2. If there is something you need to accept about yourself or others, do it now. If necessary, forgive yourself for any judgments you have been holding.

3. Let peace radiate from your heart center into the area you are working on. See the cells joyful and relaxed and thriving and revitalizing in this peaceful energy.

4. Contact your basic self by placing your hand(s) over the lower stomach area. What does your basic self indicate to you now (in words, pictures, impressions) about the imbalance or area you are looking to improve.

5. Take a moment to attune inwardly to your high self. Is there anything your high self is sharing with you?

6. Place your hands over your heart and love yourself unconditionally.

7. Create a brief self-talk/internal dialog that incorporates peace in your healing; for example, as you breathe in peace, tensions and worries drop away, and peace starts radiating through your body.

8. If there is one picture you can hold in your mind about peace that brings you to greater health and well-being, what would it be?

# Healing Stage
## 2

---

## Hope

This is a quality that is so nebulous, it's like grabbing hold of air. There is a saying, "Hope springs eternally." And that's the problem, I don't want it to keep springing up. I want it to come over here so I can do something with it. Yet the very idea that "I hope I'll get better" may be one of the stepping stones for you to start doing what is necessary for you to get healthier and come into a better and happier place. But in order to do this, you have to hope that there's a better place than where you are.

## Applying the Stages of Healing: HOPE

1. Move to your knowing that you can and will bring healing and balance to the area you are looking to improve.

2. If you have any doubts, forgive yourself for any judgments you have been holding about them.

3. Let your positive expectations for this area radiate through your body. See the cells joyful and relaxed and thriving and revitalizing in this positive, loving energy.

4. Contact your basic self by placing your hand(s) over the lower stomach area. What does your basic self indicate to you now (in words, pictures, impressions) about the imbalance or area you are looking to improve.

5. Take a moment to attune inwardly to your high self. Is there anything your high self is sharing with you?

6. Place your hands over your heart and love yourself unconditionally.

7. Create a brief self-talk/internal dialog that incorporates hope in your healing; for example, that you know you are moving into a happier and healthier place in your life.

8. If there is one picture you can hold in your mind about hope that brings you to greater health and well-being, what would it be?

# Healing Stage
## 3

_____

## JOY

*Joy, dynamically moving through your consciousness, changing, altering, updating, making all things new, is indicative of the presence of Spirit.*

Why have joy? Why not have joy? It's fun when joy comes up as a profound, ecstatic feeling. Joy comes in and you start moving with fluidity inside you, so that people can even insult you and you still have joy. You are so joyful, you are happy just to get recognized. They thought they were insulting you, and you joyfully took it as recognition. It's a wonderful feeling.

When the body, mind, and spirit are in harmony, you will experience joy along with its companion, a sense of peace.

Men and women are spiritual beings. There is nothing and no one that is not of God. The spark of God individualized within each human being is the Soul. The Soul is the basic element of our existence. The Soul is forever connected to God. That connection is perfect and intimate; it is the source from which we draw our life. The nature, the essence, of the Soul is JOY. It is joyful because it is wholly of God, is aware of that, and has total knowledge of that.

Joy, dynamically moving through your consciousness, changing, altering, updating, making all things new, is indicative of the presence of Spirit. The Spirit is always NOW, always present.

Long ago, I told myself that whenever that feeling of depression came in, it would immediately move me to joy. I reprogrammed depression for happiness. So if that feeling begins to come in, I start lifting immediately. Anything less than the "state of being" can be used to program you back into a "state of being." Anything off center can be used to move you back to center.

Anticipate joy at every moment. And always maintain a sense of gratefulness for all of your blessings. Being grateful means maintaining the awareness that Divinity is entirely present in every moment of your life and that you don't have to go anywhere to experience the glory of the divine presence. When you are in that awareness and cooperation, all things flow to you, and you experience a sense of upliftment and peace. You can turn to the positive direction at any moment, and the joy will be entirely present for you.

Joy is inherent through the Soul. When you have joy—when this happiness just comes up inside you—then no matter what you do or say or become out there, this center of calm and happiness is not disturbed because it is what it is. Therein is your fulfillment for being on this physical level.

1.  Realize that joy is present inside of you, right now.

2.  Come present with yourself right now and realize that joy is dynamically moving through your consciousness, changing, altering, updating, making all things new.

3.  Let joy radiate from your heart center into the area you are working on. See the cells joyful and relaxed and thriving and revitalizing in this joyful energy.

4.  Contact your basic self by placing your hand(s) over the lower stomach area. What does your basic self indicate to you now (in words, pictures, impressions) about the imbalance or area you are looking to improve.

5.  Take a moment to attune inwardly to your high self. Is there anything your high self is sharing with you?

6.  Place your hands over your heart and love yourself unconditionally.

7.  Create a brief self-talk/internal dialog that incorporates joy in your healing; for example, that you anticipate joy at every moment and you always maintain a sense of gratefulness for all of your blessings.

8.  If there is one picture you can hold in your mind about joy that brings you to greater health and well-being, what would it be?

# Healing Stage
## 4

_____

## FAITH

*The glory descends upon us, and we are sustained by the grace of God.*

Blind faith is not what we're dealing with here, nor faith in the biblical, religious sense. This faith is based upon something that you know you can do, which gives you the strength to take a giant step into the next thing. For example, you may say, "I don't have the faith to be a doctor." Have you gone to first year medical school? "No." Right, you don't need faith at this point; what you need is education. That education is the foundation you're building to make a step to being a doctor. And the faith is based upon evidence that you can succeed.

If I perceive grace in the experiences of my life, the wisdoms that have come forward about what to do and what not to do, then I have the trust that I can learn from my experiences, and that allows me to step onto the path of faith.

Faith is unseen substance, like air is unseen substance. We can demonstrate the existence of air as a substance by lighting incense and letting it float in the air. What is holding it up? The unseen substance.

We cannot see it, but if we put color in it (the incense smoke), we get to see what the substance is. The way we see faith is by our actions. Our actions produce the "color" in the faith, and that faith is the platform on which we step forward into nothingness, the future. The glory descends upon us, and we are sustained by the grace of God.

1. What do you know you can do in relation to the area you are balancing and healing or looking to improve?

2. Write down or say out loud an example of how grace is in your life.

3. Let the quality of faith radiate from your heart center into the area you are working on. See the cells joyful, relaxed, thriving, and revitalizing in this energy of grace.

4. Contact your basic self by placing your hand(s) over the lower stomach area. What does your basic self indicate to you now (in words, pictures, impressions) about the imbalance or area you are looking to improve.

5. Take a moment to attune inwardly to your high self. Is there anything your high self is sharing with you?

6. Place your hands over your heart and love yourself unconditionally.

7. Create a brief self-talk/internal dialog that incorporates grace in your healing; for example, that you are sustained by the grace of God.

8. If there is one picture you can hold in your mind about grace that brings you to greater health and well-being, what would it be?

# Healing Stage
# 5

---

## CERTAINTY

This certainty is a conviction deep down inside you that you are healthy, wealthy, and happy. I didn't use the word rich; I used the word wealthy in terms of being well—a state of well-being.

*You create your own hell; you create your own heaven. As a creator, it's your choice.*

What I know for certain is that who you are is beyond the body, emotions, mind, and unconscious, because you can stand back and observe those levels. What stands back and looks is the one that is the certainty. In that certainty, you know that you know despite the fact that there is no outer evidence. The evidence is revealed as you put your body on the line and live life based upon that certainty. That's why it's not called faith.

The work on this level is the love of the Soul manifesting through the physical. If you're doing a job you don't like to do, do it from the Soul, and it will be done joyfully and perfectly. If you are working with a person you don't like, look beyond the personality traits that annoy you, see the perfection of the Soul, and it'll be easy to work with that person. These things can be done—it's your choice. If you say, "I just don't understand her," you won't. If you say, "I just can't do that," you can't. You create your own reality, your own laws, out of your own divine nature. For the sake of God within you, and for the sake of God beyond you, get smart. You create your own hell; you create your own heaven. As a creator, it's your choice.

1.  Connect with the certainty that you are healthy, wealthy, and happy, right now.

2.  If there is something you need to accept about yourself or others, do it now. If necessary, forgive yourself for any judgments you have been holding.

3.  Let certainty radiate from your heart center into the area you are working on. See the cells joyful, relaxed, thriving, and revitalizing in this energy of gentle strength.

4.  Contact your basic self by placing your hand(s) over the lower stomach area. What does your basic self indicate to you now (in words, pictures, impressions) about the imbalance or area you are looking to improve.

5.  Take a moment to attune inwardly to your high self. Is there anything your high self is sharing with you?

6.  Place your hands over your heart and love yourself unconditionally.

7.  Create a brief self-talk/internal dialog that incorporates certainty in your healing; for example, that you create your own reality, your own laws, out of your own divine nature, and that you do all things from the Soul.

8.  If there is one picture you can hold in your mind about certainty that brings you to greater health and well-being, what would it be?

# Healing Stage
## 6

---

## WISDOM

When I talk about wisdom, I'm not talking about being smart. We've got smart people running the world. Look what they're doing. I'm talking about the wisdom where you are caring for yourself and the person next to you. We're talking about the wisdom of your having an experience that leads you to success. Even in the failure, you learn the success.

*Take into the body those things that will make it healthy, those things that will give it strength and beauty. That is exercising wisdom.*

It is the wisdom of experience that you are gaining here on the earth plane, and then you transfer that wisdom from point to point in this world. If other people share their experiences with you and you learn from them, you can probably cut down the time you have to sit on the borders of fear and doubt and can more quickly discover the center of your beingness and reside in the presence and joy of Spirit. Finding the "state of being" can bring you a fulfillment and a joy greater than you have ever known on this earth. It transcends all the levels of mind, emotions, and body and reaches to the inner Kingdom, wherein resides all peace, joy, and love.

When some people's marriage fails, they don't want to get married again. Yet they should be able to do the next one better and faster than the first time. So they can get in and out of it in a hurry. "I don't want to get in and out in a hurry. I want it to last." Then do those things that will make it last. Most of us know what they are. We know when to keep our mouths shut. And yet we'll say the cutting remark. That's not wisdom, that's stupid.

Use your wisdom. Do not abuse your body or corrupt it by taking into it things that will disturb or destroy the natural nerve functions. Take into the body those things that will make it healthy, those things that will give it strength and beauty. That is exercising wisdom.

Wisdom is given to all, but only a few choose to use it. If you decide you want to use your wisdom, you will get many, many chances to do so. You will discover where wisdom is. Some people think wisdom is found in the encyclopedia, the dictionary, universities, or libraries. It may be, and it may be in other books, too, or in your little son or daughter. But you will probably find that wisdom is within you because wisdom comes from God, and God is within.

There are no secrets within you. There is no solution that is hidden from you. There is nothing kept back. All wisdom is available to you at every moment, and it is your challenge and your responsibility to attune yourself to Spirit and to the God within so that you may receive the wisdom for yourself.

Wisdom is using those things that work for you, for as long as they work for you, and letting go of the things that are not working for you. Problems are beautiful because every time you handle or overcome a problem, your wisdom and your knowledge grow. Every time you overcome something, you grow. The problems give you strength to go further. Your karmic situations are your stepping-stones.

Love your karma. It is your opportunity to learn. It is your opportunity to gain wisdom.

## Applying the Stages of Healing: WISDOM

1. What guidance or counsel does your inner wisdom give you about your health and well-being?

2. Forgive yourself for any judgments you have been holding about ignoring or overriding your inner wisdom.

3. Let wisdom radiate from your heart center into the area you are working on. See the cells joyful, relaxed, thriving, and revitalizing in this beautiful energy.

4. Contact your basic self by placing your hand(s) over the lower stomach area. What does your basic self indicate to you now (in words, pictures, impressions) about the imbalance or area you are looking to improve.

5. Take a moment to attune inwardly to your high self. Is there anything your high self is sharing with you?

6. Place your hands over your heart and love yourself unconditionally.

7. Create a brief self-talk/internal dialog that incorporates wisdom in your healing; for example, that you discover the center of your beingness and reside in the presence and joy of Spirit, bringing you a fulfillment greater than you have ever known on this earth.

8. If there is one picture you can hold in your mind about wisdom that brings you to greater health and well-being, what would it be?

# Healing Stage
## 7

---

## LOVE

The love I am referring to is not inert like a bump on a log, but it is loving as an action that encompasses the other six healing stages—peace, hope, joy, faith, certainty, and wisdom. This love is where you reach out and touch someone and lift them with a smile, a look, and even with a thought. It's also saying something to them that lets them know that you care for them.

Do you know that a braggart always hears other people bragging, that the conceited person always sees conceit, that the lazy person sees laziness, and that love sees love?

Love is the essence of all creation, the "glue" that holds everything in its place in relation to all other parts and that allows it all to function. Everything is a manifestation of love, and loving is about the closest term I've come up with for the energy of Spirit.

Loving is a process that happens inside you through the grace of Spirit and by your own ability to be in touch with the God within. The loving that you have for yourself and for one another is God's love. There isn't any other love. Your loving heart is God's loving heart. Your body is God's body. The God that you are is all the other "Gods." In God, you have your living and breathing, your coming in and going out, your death and your resurrection. The whole spectrum of your life takes place within God, and anyone who is residing in the power of love is never destroyed, never separated, always free, always up, always growing.

Living love is not just loving from some place deep within you, but living love with every breath. When you breathe in, love breathes in. And when you breathe out, love breathes out. Living love also means that your love extends unconditionally to all things. You love everything present, no exceptions. Living love doesn't care whether you're black or white, female or male, drunk or sober, this or that. It is the expression of the loving heart, which knows no limitations, conditions, or restrictions. It just is—equally.

All love is within you. It's part of infinite supply; in fact, it is the infinite supply. It's important for you to keep calling forward the essence of spiritual love every day so you keep lifting higher. Let nothing stop you from this endeavor, for it is more important than any other activity.

*Love it all equally. Love it all, own it all—and you will be free.*

This physical body is truly a temple of the Spirit, for the Spirit resides in each one of us. And you can build your body so that it does not become a heavy body, but a light body, so the Spirit can work more closely with you. When you reach a harmony within you, you can take cells that have been out of balance and place a ring of love around them and hold them in balance for five, ten, fifteen years. Love and joy and happiness can change the frequency of cell structure from the "doom and gloom" of a cell disintegrating to a lilting, joyful quality of a cell lifting into balance and harmony.

Take care of yourself on all levels. Do those things that will be uplifting. Be with other people who are following the upward path. Be loving to yourself and to others. Chant the sacred names of God. Open your heart to God's presence and walk joyfully in His loving embrace.

The key to breaking free is to love yourself and to love each experience that comes to you whether it appears to be negative or positive. Love it all equally. Love it all, own it all—and you will be free.

1. What kind words do you need to say to yourself right now? Say them inwardly or out loud.

2. If there is something you have not been able to love about yourself or others, forgive yourself for any judgments you have been holding about that.

3. Let love radiate from your heart center into the area you are working on. See the cells joyful, relaxed, thriving, and revitalizing in this loving energy.

4. Contact your basic self by placing your hand(s) over the lower stomach area. What does your basic self indicate to you now (in words, pictures, impressions) about the imbalance or area you are looking to improve.

5. Take a moment to attune inwardly to your high self. Is there anything your high self is sharing with you?

6. Place your hands over your heart and love yourself unconditionally.

7. Create a brief self-talk/internal dialog that incorporates love in your healing; for example, that you open your heart to God's presence and walk joyfully in His loving embrace.

8. If there is one picture you can hold in your mind about love that brings you to greater health and well-being, what would it be?

# A 30-Day Program

For Your Health and Well-Being

Now that you have read the book, you may choose to create your own health program. Here is a 30-day program of discovery that you can use as a springboard into greater health and well-being for the rest of your life. You will need a journal.

Consider making your journal a creative experience, using colored pencils, relevant clippings from magazines—such as pictures, images, and cut-out words or phrases. You can also trace or photocopy pictures and images from books, or have images on your computer screen as an inspiration.

It is recommended that you keep a journal of one or more of the following:

1) What and how much you eat.

2) Your methods for moving your body—yoga, tai chi, jogging, walking, etc.

3) Your inner work—meditation, breathing practice, spiritual exercises.

4) Your sleep patterns—when you go to bed, when you rise, how much sleep you get.

Before beginning the program, you may want to take time to set up your journal or tracking system.

Feel free to tailor this program to your own personal needs, keeping in mind two keys: do something positive for your health and well-being and do it consistently. You'll have noticed that a continual theme throughout this book is loving. So your 30-day program could be as simple as taking a few moments each day to love your body and love every aspect of yourself. Such moments can be found while waiting at a stop light or in line at the supermarket checkout. There is always an opportunity to relax, breathe, and bathe all the cells of your body in Light and love.

As you work on the questions or direction for each day, remember to call in the Light *(see page 161)* for the highest good.

# Day One:
_____

One of the goals of the book (other than giving you choices on how you can direct your health and well-being) is to make one small, significant, meaningful step towards your health and well-being that can be sustained and maintained for the rest of your life.

What is the small step you have in mind?

It could be something you are adding, for example, walking for 20 minutes, three times a week, or meditating for 5 minutes a day. Or it could be something you are taking away—like reducing your sugar intake.

Whatever it is, keep it in mind as you go through these 30 days. There is no need to commit to anything now, though you may want to try it on for size in the meantime. The exercises over the next 30 days will assist you to find clarity. The conclusion of the 30 days will be the time to commit to your direction towards greater health.

# Day Two:

_____

Choose an area of health that is an issue or problem for you or an area that you wish to improve or make better.

As you write about this area, be as specific and as detailed as you can.

What do you know to do that you are not doing in this area? Again, be as detailed and specific as you can.

Read what you have written. Forgive yourself for any judgments that may have arisen.

# Day Three:

_____

Keeping in mind the area you chose in Day Two, what are you doing that you know not to do in this area?

As you write about this area, be as specific and as detailed as you can.

Read what you have written. Forgive yourself for any judgments that may have arisen.

# Day Four:

_____

Write your story about what happened in regard to what you have described on Day Two and Day Three.

What philosophy have you developed to support your behaving contrary to what you know?

As you write the answer, be as detailed as you can, bringing in your childhood, parents, upbringing, religion, beliefs, life experience, etc., where appropriate.

# Day Five:

_____

As you review the story you wrote on Day Four, what consistent theme emerges out of the story?

Pay particular attention to, and write about, when you felt you were a victim.

Also pay attention to, and describe, the judgments you made—and perhaps are still presently making—on yourself, others, the world, God, etc.

# Day Six:

_____

Review what you wrote on Day Five.

Close your eyes and place you hand (or hands) over the basic self area in your lower abdomen. Extend your loving through your hands into this area.

Ask the basic self to please communicate with you, at this time, about how you can improve your health and well-being in the area that you are working with *(see Day Two)*.

Write down what you see or hear, or receive intuitively.

Take some time, now, to forgive yourself for the judgments you have made on yourself, others, the world, God, etc. Do this out loud. (See appendix on Forgiveness, for how to forgive yourself.)

When complete, close your eyes and take a moment to focus on your breathing—the gentle rising and falling of your breath. This will bring you into a relaxed and calm place inside yourself.

Feel the presence of Light and love.

# Day Seven:

"When the conscious self asserts its will, it is really quite powerful. But in a showdown of willpower with the basic self, nine times out of ten, the basic will win. But when it comes to using the imagination, nine times out of ten, the conscious self will win, because the basic can only accept what consciousness places in it. So if you maintain a positive image of completion, the basic self will accept it and work with it. If you place an image forward, the basic sees it and goes to work to make it come about; it asserts energy into those levels to bring it about."

Please take time to contemplate this important quote from the book throughout this day.

It's vital that you not underestimate the power of your own images and thoughts and how you can work with them for your greater health and well-being.

# Day Eight:

_____

Keeping in mind the area you have chosen to work on, now ask for the highest good as you attune inwardly to your High Self.

Is there any guidance your High Self is sharing with you at this time?

Be sensitive to words, images, or your own intuition that you may receive.

Write these down and review them before you go to bed this evening. Before going to sleep, keeping in mind the highest good of all concerned, ask that you be given guidance towards better health and well-being in ways that you understand.

Also, before going to sleep, take some time to forgive yourself for any judgments you have placed on yourself, on others, on the world, on God, etc. Do this out loud, if you can.

# Day Nine:

_____

Once again reviewing the area of health and well-being you are working on now, write a new story—a story of success in the area you are working on.

Describe in detail your approach and attitude and the successful outcome in this area.

Bring in how you feel in your body, your emotional state, what you are thinking, and the level of loving you are giving yourself. This is your story of expansion.

When you are complete with writing, put your pen and journal down and begin to focus on your breathing—the rising and falling of your breath.

Let your breath bring you into a relaxed and calm place inside yourself. Close your eyes and take in what you have just learned. Fill yourself with the positive imagery you have just elucidated in your journal.

# Day Ten:

_____

In the last few days, you have had a wonderful look at the direction you want to go in relation to your health and well-being. Now that you are clear, it's time to let go of what might be coming between you and having greater health.

If you have not been doing free-form writing, this is an excellent time to start the practice. It is perhaps the best tool around for clearing the unconscious levels.

Review the chapter on free-form writing on page 243. Find a quiet time and place and begin your practice. Commit to a minimum of 15 minutes a day. It's best to set a timer or alarm. That way you can fully give yourself to the process without distraction.

# Day Eleven:

_____

Continue with your free-form writing.

Everyone is looking for the "magic bullet," the one thing or remedy that will solve or prevent all of our health problems. However, there is one remedy that comes closest to this ideal—exercise.

You really must move your body, every day, even if it is a short walk. What exercise or movement practice can you do every day for a minimum of ten minutes? You can vary it if you wish—walking one day, yoga another, etc.

# Day Twelve:

_____

Continue with your free-form writing (minimum 15 minutes).

Continue with your exercise activity (minimum 10 minutes).

It's very well documented that the United States is a sleep-deprived nation. If you have not been tracking your sleep patterns, it would be a very good idea to begin to do so. Better rest means better and clearer decisions. It also means a stronger immune system and better protection against diabetes.

Each person varies as to what is the optimum amount of sleep. Your level of wellness will also be a big factor in this. However, eight hours remains a good guideline with many people needing more and many able to get by quite well on less.

# Day Thirteen:

_____

Continue with your free-form writing (minimum 15 minutes).

Continue with your exercise activity (minimum 10 minutes).

Continue to track your sleep patterns and monitor that you are getting enough rest.

In the section on *Applying the Principles* on page 73, which area has the greatest opportunity for improvement? Less stress, less sugar, or less acid?

Write down a small step you can take in the area you have chosen.

# Day Fourteen:

_____

Continue with your free-form writing (minimum 15 minutes).

Continue with your exercise activity (minimum 10 minutes).

Continue to track your sleep patterns and monitor that you are getting enough rest.

Continue to take a small step in applying the principles.

Using your knowledge of yourself, your intuition, or through self muscle-testing, find an area in the section on _Causes and Cures of Disease_, page 103, that has meaning and resonance for you.

Write your story about how this area (the cause and/or the cure) impacts your life. Be as detailed as you can, bringing in your childhood, parents, upbringing, religion, beliefs, life experience, etc., where appropriate.

# Day Fifteen:

Regarding yesterday's exercise on the causes and cures of disease, contact your basic self by placing your hand(s) over the lower stomach area. What does your basic self indicate to you (perhaps by words, pictures, impressions)?

Perhaps your basic self has a different story or perspective than the one you just wrote above, in which case let the basic self speak and give its story. Write down what you hear or perceive it to say.

Forgive yourself out loud for any judgments that have surfaced or are present.

What's the next step that you see for yourself in the area you described?

Continue with your free-form writing (minimum 15 minutes).

Continue with your exercise activity (minimum 10 minutes).

Continue to track your sleep patterns and monitor that you are getting enough rest.

Continue to take a small step in applying the principles.

# Day Sixteen:

_____

Keeping in mind the area of health you are looking to improve, and also keeping in mind yesterday's exercise, take a moment to attune inwardly to your high self.

Is there anything your high self is sharing with you through your intuition—in words, pictures, or symbols?

Write down your impressions, even if it seems you are making them up. (There is a reason you are making up what you are writing rather than making up something else.)

Take a moment to appreciate the way that your basic self, your conscious self, and your high self are working together. When they work in harmony, it is a spiritual marriage.

Continue with your free-form writing (minimum 15 minutes).

Continue with your exercise activity (minimum 10 minutes).

Continue to track your sleep patterns and monitor that you are getting enough rest.

Continue to take a small step in applying the principles.

# Day Seventeen:

Review the section on healing sound, on page 175. Choose a sound that works for you and incorporate it into a daily, five-minute practice—for example, just before or just after you exercise.

Continue with your free-form writing (minimum 15 minutes).

Continue with your exercise activity (minimum 10 minutes).

Continue to track your sleep patterns and monitor that you are getting enough rest.

Continue to take a small step in applying the principles.

# Day Eighteen:

_____

Review your story of success on Day Nine. Incorporate this into a brief script of your new self-talk (see page 49 on self talk).

As you write this script, be sure to incorporate its multi-dimensional elements and components.

The physical element—what it looks like.

The emotional element—what it feels like.

The mental element—what you think about it.

The spiritual element—the higher perspective.

Continue with your free-form writing (minimum 15 minutes).

Continue with your exercise activity (minimum 10 minutes).

Continue to track your sleep patterns and monitor that you are getting enough rest.

Continue to take a small step in applying the principles.

Continue to practice a healing sound (minimum 5 minutes).

# Day Nineteen:

_____

Read your self-talk script for your health and well-being. Try it on for size. See how it fits you and make any adjustments.

You are going to read it to yourself, preferably out loud, at least once a day.

Continue with your free-form writing (minimum 15 minutes).

Continue with your exercise activity (minimum 10 minutes).

Continue to track your sleep patterns and monitor that you are getting enough rest.

Continue to take a small step in applying the principles.

Continue to practice a healing sound (minimum 5 minutes).

# Day Twenty:

---

Re-read the chapter on the principle of holding the pictures in your mind that you want more of *(page 23)*.

What pictures come to mind that you want more of?

Can you envision them clearly?

Are they reflected in the pictures from magazines and books that you have cut out, traced, or photocopied for your journal? If not, choose a way to find pictures and images that inspire you.

Start a daily practice of envisioning clearly your improved health and well-being so it becomes a habit.

Continue with your free-form writing (minimum 15 minutes).

Continue with your exercise activity (minimum 10 minutes).

Continue to track your sleep patterns and monitor that you are getting enough rest.

Continue to take a small step in applying the principles.

Continue to practice a healing sound (minimum 5 minutes).

Read your self-talk script at least once a day.

# Day Twenty-one:

Using your knowledge of yourself, your intuition, or through self muscle-testing, find another area in the section on *Causes and Cures of Disease*, page 103, that has meaning and resonance for you. In choosing this area, ask yourself what is the single most important, effective thing that you can do to improve your health and well-being? In other words, if there was just one thing you could do, what would it be? Write down what you come up with.

Write your story about how this area (the cause and/or the cure) impacts your life. Be as detailed as you can, bringing in your childhood, parents, upbringing, religion, beliefs, life experience, etc., where appropriate. There is no need to repeat what you wrote on Day Fourteen, but do see if you can go a little deeper or find a new twist or nuance.

Continue with your free-form writing (minimum 15 minutes).

Continue with your exercise activity (minimum 10 minutes).

Continue to track your sleep patterns and monitor that you are getting enough rest.

Continue to take a small step in applying the principles.

Continue to practice a healing sound (minimum 5 minutes).

Read your self-talk script at least once a day.

Envision the pictures of health and well-being that you have chosen as wanting more of.

# Day Twenty-two:

_____

Regarding yesterday's exercise on the causes and cures of disease, contact your basic self by placing your hand(s) over the lower stomach area. What does your basic self indicate to you (perhaps by words, pictures, impressions)?

Perhaps your basic self has a different story or perspective than the one you wrote yesterday, in which case let the basic self speak and give its story. Write down what you hear or perceive it to say.

Forgive yourself out loud for any judgments that have surfaced or are present.

What's the next step that you see for yourself in the area you described?

Continue with your free-form writing (minimum 15 minutes).

Continue with your exercise activity (minimum 10 minutes).

Continue to track your sleep patterns and monitor that you are getting enough rest.

Continue to take a small step in applying the principles.

Continue to practice a healing sound (minimum 5 minutes).

Read your self-talk script at least once a day.

Envision the pictures of health and well-being that you have chosen as wanting more of.

# Day Twenty-three:

_____

Keeping in mind the area of health you are looking to improve, and also keeping in mind yesterday's exercise, take a moment to attune inwardly to your high self.

Is there anything your high self is sharing with you through your intuition—in words, pictures, or symbols?

Write down your impressions, even if it seems you are making them up. (There is a reason you are making up what you are writing rather than making up something else.)

Take a moment to appreciate the way that your basic self, your conscious self, and your high self are working together. When they work in harmony, it is a spiritual marriage.

Continue with your free-form writing (minimum 15 minutes).

Continue with your exercise activity (minimum 10 minutes).

Continue to track your sleep patterns and monitor that you are getting enough rest.

Continue to take a small step in applying the principles.

Continue to practice a healing sound (minimum 5 minutes).

Read your self-talk script at least once a day.

Envision the pictures of health and well-being that you have chosen as wanting more of.

# Day Twenty-four:

_____

It's now time to take the key area of imbalance that you have been working on through the healing stages, beginning on page 189.

As you go through the healing stage of PEACE, write down what is going on inside you as your area of imbalance is being transformed, healed, and made whole.

At any time, forgive yourself, preferably out loud, for any judgments that surface.

When you have gone through all this healing stage, spend a few moments of quiet taking it in.

Write what you are experiencing.

Continue with your free-form writing (minimum 15 minutes).

Continue with your exercise activity (minimum 10 minutes).

Continue to track your sleep patterns and monitor that you are getting enough rest.

Continue to take a small step in applying the principles.

Continue to practice a healing sound (minimum 5 minutes).

Read your self-talk script at least once a day.

Envision the pictures of health and well-being that you have chosen as wanting more of.

# Day Twenty-five:

_____

As you go through the healing stage of HOPE, write down what is going on inside you as your area of imbalance is being transformed, healed, and made whole.

At any time, forgive yourself, preferably out loud, for any judgments that surface.

When you have gone through all this healing stage, spend a few moments of quiet taking it in.

Write what you are experiencing.

Continue with your free-form writing (minimum 15 minutes).

Continue with your exercise activity (minimum 10 minutes).

Continue to track your sleep patterns and monitor that you are getting enough rest.

Continue to take a small step in applying the principles.

Continue to practice a healing sound (minimum 5 minutes).

Read your self-talk script at least once a day.

Envision the pictures of health and well-being that you have chosen as wanting more of.

# Day Twenty-six:

As you go through the healing stage of JOY, write down what is going on inside you as your area of imbalance is being transformed, healed, and made whole.

At any time, forgive yourself, preferably out loud, for any judgments that surface.

When you have gone through all this healing stage, spend a few moments of quiet taking it in.

Write what you are experiencing.

Continue with your free-form writing (minimum 15 minutes).

Continue with your exercise activity (minimum 10 minutes).

Continue to track your sleep patterns and monitor that you are getting enough rest.

Continue to take a small step in applying the principles.

Continue to practice a healing sound (minimum 5 minutes).

Read your self-talk script at least once a day.

Envision the pictures of health and well-being that you have chosen as wanting more of.

# Day Twenty-seven:

_____

As you go through the healing stage of FAITH, write down what is going on inside you as your area of imbalance is being transformed, healed, and made whole.

At any time, forgive yourself, preferably out loud, for any judgments that surface.

When you have gone through all this healing stage, spend a few moments of quiet taking it in.

Write what you are experiencing.

Continue with your free-form writing (minimum 15 minutes).

Continue with your exercise activity (minimum 10 minutes).

Continue to track your sleep patterns and monitor that you are getting enough rest.

Continue to take a small step in applying the principles.

Continue to practice a healing sound (minimum 5 minutes).

Read your self-talk script at least once a day.

Envision the pictures of health and well-being that you have chosen as wanting more of.

# Day Twenty-eight:
_____

As you go through the healing stage of CERTAINTY, write down what is going on inside you as your area of imbalance is being transformed, healed, and made whole.

At any time, forgive yourself, preferably out loud, for any judgments that surface.

When you have gone through all this healing stage, spend a few moments of quiet taking it in.

Write what you are experiencing.

Continue with your free-form writing (minimum 15 minutes).

Continue with your exercise activity (minimum 10 minutes).

Continue to track your sleep patterns and monitor that you are getting enough rest.

Continue to take a small step in applying the principles.

Continue to practice a healing sound (minimum 5 minutes).

Read your self-talk script at least once a day.

Envision the pictures of health and well-being that you have chosen as wanting more of.

# Day Twenty-nine:

As you go through the healing stage of WISDOM, write down what is going on inside you as your area of imbalance is being transformed, healed, and made whole.

At any time, forgive yourself, preferably out loud, for any judgments that surface.

When you have gone through all this healing stage, spend a few moments of quiet taking it in.

Write what you are experiencing.

Continue with your free-form writing (minimum 15 minutes).

Continue with your exercise activity (minimum 10 minutes).

Continue to track your sleep patterns and monitor that you are getting enough rest.

Continue to take a small step in applying the principles.

Continue to practice a healing sound (minimum 5 minutes).

Read your self-talk script at least once a day.

Envision the pictures of health and well-being that you have chosen as wanting more of.

# Day Thirty:

_____

As you go through the healing stage of LOVE, write down what is going on inside you as your area of imbalance is being transformed, healed, and made whole.

At any time, forgive yourself, preferably out loud, for any judgments that surface.

When you have gone through all this healing stage, spend a few moments of quiet taking it in.

Write what you are experiencing.

Continue with your free-form writing (minimum 15 minutes).

Continue with your exercise activity (minimum 10 minutes).

Continue to track your sleep patterns and monitor that you are getting enough rest.

Continue to take a small step in applying the principles.

Continue to practice a healing sound (minimum 5 minutes).

Read your self-talk script at least once a day.

Envision the pictures of health and well-being that you have chosen as wanting more of.

You have now completed your 30-day program. Congratulations.

Your health is now in your hands. Use what you know. And always apply it using the measure of common sense, taking care of yourself so you can help take care of others; not hurting yourself and not hurting others; and using everything for your upliftment, learning, and growth.

If you can take one small thing you learned from this book and apply it consistently, you will understand how you can naturally build good habit patterns for your health and well-being.

Perhaps you may want to continue to keep a daily health journal so that you can be vigilant with your health and maintain your newly developed good habits.

# Appendix

Free-Form Writing
Forgiveness
Spiritual Exercises
Interview with John-Roger (1984)

# Free-Form Writing

Negative elements that lodge in our unconscious and subconscious levels are difficult to clear because, by definition, these levels are not conscious. We create these elements by repressing things, by obsessing, and by being "possessed" by such things as smoking, alcohol, and food. Doing free-form writing is especially helpful for clearing this kind of negative influence, and it may be the most valuable thing you learn from this book.

The unconscious is one of our most powerful influences because, by its very nature, we cannot be aware of its influence until it surfaces. We may find ourselves thinking, feeling, and doing things that we cannot explain or experiencing illness or pain with an unknown cause. The vastness of the unconscious is impossible to fully explore. It marks the division between our waking awareness and our true spiritual nature, and to become aware of our Soul, we have to cross that line into the unconscious. As we do so, we lose something of our daylight awareness. That is why so many people talk about their spiritual nature but so few are aware of it as a living experience.

For years, I have used free-form writing to help clear my unconscious. It is very simple to do. I have described in the next few pages the way I approach it, a way that I know works.

**1.** Find a quiet place and sit down with a ballpoint pen and paper. I also recommend that you light a candle because as you write, emotional negativity may come up and release into the room. Since it tends to go towards flame, having a lit candle may keep the room clear and the negativity away from you.

**2.** Allow a thought into your mind and transfer it into the pen and onto the paper. You may not even finish a sentence before the next thought comes up. For example, the thought "go to the restaurant together" arises. As you write "go to the," you may have another thought, so you start to write that next thought. You do not need to finish the first one. The next word or thought that comes up may be "help," and you may write "hlp." That is fine because you know what you mean by it and you do not have to worry about spelling (or punctuation). But do not write in shorthand because that was not the form through which the thoughts and images lodged in your subconscious or unconscious.

It is important that you do not do free-form writing on a computer or a typewriter, since typing it does not carry the same impact and there may be too much negative energy releasing for the typewriter or computer to handle. Also, do not do free-form writing on a chalkboard or white board and then erase it. The energy that you released may stay in the board itself.

Free-form writing is a kinesthetic activity. The neural impulses from the fingers are sent back to the brain so that the writing actually releases and records the patterns of the unconscious. I call them the "beach balls," those things we have suppressed for a long, long time and on which we have expended energy to keep under the surface. They can carry tremendous emotion. So at times you may end up writing very forcefully. That's why I recommend that you do not write with a pencil: the lead can break and you lose the flow.

In some instances, you will find yourself writing as fast as you can, and at other times you will be writing slowly. But throughout this process, you should be writing continuously because there are always thoughts in your mind–and you are to write them down, even if they are, "I don't know why I'm doing this. What should I write next? Hmmmm." And do not be concerned if only "junk" is coming up when you do free-form writing; this means that the free-form writing is working.

It is very important when doing free-form writing that you do not just let the pen write. That is automatic writing, a very different process, in which you may be giving over your consciousness to something outside of yourself. Free-form writing is stream-of-consciousness writing, where you just write whatever comes into your mind. You are not giving yourself over to anything in this process because you are in absolute control of what is happening. You also write with the hand that you normally write with, not your other hand; free-form writing is different from the technique of writing with the subdominant hand.

**3.** When you get through writing, do not read it over. Rip up what you have written and either burn it or flush it down the toilet. Some people still feel the energy of what they have released even after they have burned (or flushed) the paper on which they did the free-form writing. It is important that you stop the process when you stop writing. Have a set amount of time to write, and when it is over, get up right away (mid-word if necessary), drink some water, move around, burn or flush what you have written right afterwards, and go on with something else. Also, do not go back in your mind to what you wrote or anything you went through or felt when you wrote it. Let it all go.

If you keep the paper, the lower levels of consciousness will hold on to the pattern, and the release will not happen. For the lower consciousness or the subconscious to release and let go of the things it has expressed, that paper must be destroyed. And after you have burned or flushed it, fill the empty space where the images and words were with loving and God. Do spiritual exercises, and allow the healing and the peace of Spirit to fill you.

After you have done free-form writing for any length of time, you may start to get some beautiful, inspirational, wonderful prose that you may want to keep, but when you are through with your session, you may forget where the beautiful writing was and want to read through what you wrote to find it. Do not do this because the energy and negativity that you released onto the paper can return to you if you reread it. Instead, as you are writing and thoughts are flowing through, take the pieces of paper on which you write the inspirational thoughts and set them aside, separate from the other writing. When you finish your session, rewrite the sections you want to keep. Then you can rip up and burn or flush all the original pages.

**4.** Never share what you have written with anyone else. If necessary, lock your door while you do free-form writing. If someone knocks, do not feel obligated to answer. You can tell people, "If my door is locked and it says, 'Do not disturb,' stay away. I will probably be out in a couple of hours."

**5.** Start slowly, but work up to writing for at least an hour. Actually, two hours per session of free-form writing is optimal. Each person is different, but to notice some real changes, I recommend doing free-form writing for a minimum of three times a week for a minimum of three months. With practice, you can get to the point where you can do this in fifteen minutes, but it will probably take you a year or so to get to that point. You can start by doing fifteen minutes at a time; then increase it, the idea being to work up to sessions of one or two hours. Don't let the fact that two hours is optimal get in your way. As with anything I suggest, try it out as best you can.

The first time people approach this, they usually sit down and think, "I wonder what I should write." Instead, they should be writing, "I wonder what I should write… Gee, this sure is stupid… I think this makes me look like a fool… I feel like such a phony… run… can't…yes… the green elephant was there… no… the cows jumped… I can't… I don't know why I'm doing it." You will see a flow begin, and then all of a sudden it may become jumbled. You may think, "I wonder why I wrote 'green elephant.'" Don't start doing that. Instead, write, "I wonder why I wrote green elephant." The writing will open the mind again, and the repository of jumbled information that has been holding energy will start to release.

## The Effects of Free-Form Writing

As you do this technique, a wonderful thing can take place. Because your free-form writing is often a symbol of an inner disturbance, you may find that pressure leaves you as you write. Obsessive behavior or habitual patterns may suddenly disappear, and you won't even know what it was that was inside you or how it managed to get there. You will just know that it is gone. Often, it will feel like relief or a sense that somebody has taken a weight off you. The strange thing is that you will probably not be aware that it was there until it is gone. Such is the nature of the unconscious.

When it goes, I would strongly advise that you not even question what it was because you might find it and reestablish it inside. We are powerful creators. Just by thinking about how glad you are to be rid of it, you could reactivate your own memory of it and—poof!—it's in.

I emphasize this because it is very hard to get something out a second time. I am speaking from personal experience. I once relooked at something, and it took me fifteen years before I was able to clear it again. I was aware every day that I had not cleared it, so I just kept at it. And one day it went. I knew what it was when it released because of where it was expressing in my body. And I just smiled and got busy doing something else to distract my mind so I would not go back to see if I had really released it.

There is something crazy about our human minds. We say, "But is it really gone?" And in doing so, we can bring it back. It is as if we were to quit smoking and then smoke another cigarette just to see if we really quit. Then we are hooked again. My advice is that when you let anything go, do not be concerned about it. Just let it go.

I have seen some phenomenal things occur with free-form writing; it has released people from psychologically restrictive patterns and from physical and emotional pain. Free-form writing does not do a great deal for you spiritually, but if you are feeling clearer and better about yourself, there is a very good chance you will feel better about doing spiritual exercises, which will do things for you spiritually. With your unconscious free, you will be in a better position to be aware of your Spirit. As a stepping-stone to Soul awareness, free-form writing is wonderful.

When I see people grieving over the death of their loved ones, I can get drawn into it in negative ways. So I will spend a lot of time writing to free myself from this restriction. You can have a tremendous amount of empathy for others without letting their grief drag you under.

Free-form writing is like taking an onion and cutting a wedge through to the center. Then you leave a space, cut another wedge, and so on. If you leave the onion exposed to the air after cutting several wedges and do no more, the sections of onion that were between the wedges will dry up and peel away. And after a time there will be just a tiny seed left. In the same way, by releasing some disturbances through free-form writing, others still inside you will fall away.

When, after free-form writing, you realize that you had been carrying excessive weight or baggage, rejoice in the feeling of freedom. When something releases, immediately stand up, stretch, and move around physically to experience your new freedom. If you let the area get rigid and tense, you may have another problem to deal with. You will often feel a sense of diminishment taking place, as though you are moving backwards inside yourself, away from things; they are getting smaller and smaller as you move back. Don't be disturbed. That just means that you are moving away from the materiality of the world.

# Forgiveness

Forgiving ourselves certainly seems to go against the grain of our human conditioning. Even the idea can bring up feelings of unworthiness or skepticism that it could possibly work. Yet if we recognize that we are, indeed, divine beings made in God's image, the idea does not seem too far-fetched, and as we look at life from that higher perspective, the idea of holding onto judgments and seeking revenge or retribution begins to seem the far odder approach.

Forgiveness points us back to ourselves as sacred, spiritual beings who have been given the gift of creation. We can use this gift to create positively or negatively. Often, when we see our negative creation or its consequences—for example, when we have gotten angry and have hurt the feelings of someone we love—it is easy to feel bad and to judge our action and ourselves. Unfortunately, that type of approach only compounds the negativity.

*Forgiveness points us back to ourselves as sacred, spiritual beings who have been given the gift of creation.*

Punishing ourselves in an attempt to balance the action through the law of "an eye for an eye and a tooth for a tooth" is a lower path. Forgiveness is the higher road. It is the road on which we walk under grace. And it is this road that has been prepared for us by the great spiritual masters who have come forward and demonstrated the consciousness of the Christ.

How, then, do you forgive yourself? The first thing you can do is simply say, "I forgive myself." Then just let go of what is bothering you. If you wish, you can add, "I let this go into the Light, for the highest good," or "I give this to God."

How do you know if you have really let it go? You may find yourself taking a deep breath, you may experience a lightness, or you may just feel better inside. Then again, you may feel nothing at all. This does not mean that nothing has happened; however, if you still sense the presence of the imbalance or negativity, it could be that you need to be more specific or precise in your forgiveness.

For example, you can say, "I forgive myself for judging my father for not giving me the love I wanted," or "I forgive myself for judging myself for not feeling worthy of my parents' love." Feel free to keep trying out lots of possibilities, and it really helps to be sincere, honest, and direct with yourself.

Notice that each phrase starts with "I forgive myself." This is because we are taking responsibility for the negativity or imbalance we have been holding onto. We can say that we forgive the other person, but, in reality, they have already been forgiven by God, so it isn't necessary. God has already forgiven us, too, but if we are still carrying the weight of the negativity, it is then necessary to forgive ourselves.

Even though the person we have judged may no longer be in our lives, or may even be dead, we still may be carrying them inside ourselves as less than the divine being they are. So it is inside that we must bring ourselves to peace with them, and forgiveness is one of the most effective ways of doing that.

Before going to sleep at night, it is nice to quickly review the day and forgive yourself for anything that is still on your mind or troubling you. And you can also do this throughout the day, whenever you notice yourself judging, so that you can live in a constant state of forgiveness.

Sometimes, however, we don't want to forgive ourselves, or we are so cut off from our loving that we don't know where to start. The basic thing we need to do is to forgive ourselves for forgetting that we are divine. That is the real message to open up the channel for our return to the Spirit.

God is in the business of forgiveness. As I have looked at life on this planet, I have often thought that perhaps our job is to make sure that God stays in business. Then again, perhaps God put us here because He wanted His children to get the necessary training so that they could all go into His business.

# Spiritual Exercises

There is one thing you can do here physically that can improve your ability to consciously know the reality of your existence on the higher spiritual levels, and that is spiritual exercises. S.e.'s are designed exactly for that purpose. They can also help you anchor into your physical body the unconditional loving and blessings that God has for you.

S.e.'s are an active technique of holding the mind steady and quieting the emotions by using a spiritual tone or vibration to connect to the energy that flows from God throughout all existence. Doing s.e.'s can help you transcend illusions and limitations and move into the awareness of Soul.

*Soul and Spirit are active, and it takes an active process to move into the Soul, which is why I teach spiritual exercises.*

When you pray you ask God, when you meditate you listen, and when you contemplate you think about what you heard and how you are going to work that. Soul and Spirit are active, and it takes an active process to move into the Soul, which is why I teach spiritual exercises. This is the one that goes through the heavens into the Kingdom of God, while the other three take you only into the Kingdom of Heaven.

In MSIA, there are a number of tones that we chant during s.e.'s. The two main ones that are good to start with are HU and ANI-HU, which are explained in pages 179 and 180. HU is the ultimate highest sound.

Spirit motivates all things. The Sound created by the Spirit in its movement is the two tones H and U. These two tones, one positive and one negative, encompass every tone and every sound that exist in the universe. When you combine them into one tone—HU—that tone is within all other tones. In this new dispensation, mankind is moving increasingly into the heritage of the HU-man; each person is becoming the God-man.

If you have misunderstanding within yourself or with someone else, you would probably want to work with the ANI-HU. If we could really know what is in the hearts of our "enemies," we would never do another thing to hurt them because there is already enough hurt. All we do is stand back and love them. The ANI-HU can give us this compassion.

These tones open the centers in the head. In MSIA, we do not work in any level below the upper part of the third eye. This is not because the energy of the centers below that is "bad" but because the most direct path to Soul Transcendence is through the top two centers. The lower centers can take a person through many, many distractions. For example, they can make you feel very lusty. You can be led astray, and it is important to be careful.

Chanting HU or ANI-HU, builds a bridge (opens a channel) between your consciousness and the higher consciousness. You may not walk across the bridge immediately because you may not have it solid enough. Let's say you have done spiritual exercises for three weeks, two hours a day, and nothing has happened. Then you may be walking down the street and a flash of insight comes in. Now, how do you think you got that? You went across the bridge.

The main thing to keep in mind when doing s.e.'s is that the only wrong way to do s.e.'s is not to do them. Perhaps the easiest way to do s.e.'s is simply to be open to receive whatever is there for you at the time. You can call in the Light and ask to become attuned to the Mystical Traveler within you, and then chant HU or ANI-HU, or your initiation tone. If you are new to s.e.'s, you might do this for ten minutes a day, more if you like, of course.

More important than the time you spend doing s.e.'s is having an attitude of "Lord, I am open to receive from you." And above all, s.e.'s are an action of the heart. So do what you can to bring forward the devotion that brought you to want to know more about God and the Divine in you. One of the great values of spiritual exercises is that they give you a chance to attune yourself to the Spirit inside you and become aware, once again, of the loving that is extended to you through Christ. All you have to do is follow the loving back into the heart of God, your home in Spirit.

Worshiping God is worthwhile. We call it doing spiritual exercises. People get astounded when they realize that by doing spiritual exercises, they have been worshiping God with their body, mind, and Soul.

## How To Do Spiritual Exercises

The only wrong way to do s.e.'s is not to do them, and there is no required way to do s.e.'s. For people who would like to have some form of methodology, here is a step-by-step procedure as a suggestion for doing fifteen minutes of s.e.'s.

1.  Find a quiet place with low lighting and a comfortable chair to sit in. It is best not to listen to music while doing s.e.'s, although it is fine to listen to music while getting ready to start.

2.  Sit upright, if possible, and close your eyes.

3.  Call yourself forward into the Light for the highest good, and ask for spiritual protection and guidance during your s.e.'s.

Take all the loving energy that has been extended into you and around you and through you, and slowly pull it up through your body until it gathers behind your eyes in the center of your forehead. Hold your attention there. Your spirit rises. The world is forgotten, and you begin your journey with the Traveler into the higher realms of Spirit.

4.  Chant HU or ANI-HU. It is preferable to do this inwardly (silently). If you are an initiate, you would chant your initiation tone.

5.  While chanting, focus your attention in the area near the center of the head directly back from your forehead. This is called the tisra til, and it is in this place that the Soul has its seat and the Soul energy gathers.

6. After you have chanted for about five minutes, stop and listen within. You are listening for the Sound Current, which is very subtle. You may hear it the first time you do this, or it may take years of practice. It is a very individual matter.

7. If you find your mind wandering and you lose the focus of listening, you can focus the mind by chanting again.

8. After about five minutes of listening, you can either continue to listen and look inside or return to chanting again. The times are approximate, of course. The idea is to spend time in s.e.'s doing both chanting and listening.

9. If you see the color purple coming from the right or center of your head, you can allow yourself to follow this inwardly, for this is a form the Mystical Traveler often takes. If the color (or any other form) is coming from the left side, we advise not following it because this is often a negative influence. (All this applies to seeing inwardly.)

10. After about five minutes, you can open your eyes. You may want to wiggle your fingers and toes to bring the energy back into your physical body. And so ends your fifteen minute session of s.e.'s.

    For longer periods of s.e.'s, you can expand the time for chanting and listening to fifteen minutes each. For example, in an hour session of s.e.'s, you can chant for fifteen minutes, listen for fifteen minutes, and then repeat the chanting-and-listening cycle.

All the above are guidelines, and it's important to remember that the only wrong way to do s.e.'s is not to do them. So you can experiment with how you do s.e.'s, using what works for you at a particular time and not getting attached to a certain form. And again, the focus is on doing your spiritual exercises with as much loving and devotion to God as you can.

# An Interview with John-Roger

*This interview was given to* The Movement Newspaper *(now* The New Day Herald, *www.newdayherald.com) on February 13, 1984.*

**MOVEMENT NEWSPAPER:  People ask you a lot of questions about their health. What do most people seem to be concerned with?**

**JOHN-ROGER:** I think that mostly they're afraid of dying. Their concern about their health is really concern about dying. If they could deal with their fear of dying then they would probably deal much better with their health.

**MN:  Even if I get a cold?**

**J-R:** People's real concerns about health are related to more serious illnesses and diseases. I'm of the persuasion that having a cold is a symptom of cleansing the body. The cure for the cold is to have a healthy body—not to try to cure the cold because the cold is already a curing device, a cleansing of the body. I call things like colds transient problems. You really can't hang onto a cold for too long. It finally tires of you and leaves. Or, you come into balance and then it leaves.

**MN:  Are colds usually emotionally related?**

**J-R:** You can get a cold from being out in the rain and getting a chill in the body, or from eating the wrong kinds of foods for you. But there are feelings that go with words. Certain words have more emotional content than others. If I use those words and place additional drama on them, intensifying them and yelling them at you, that can shake up your subtle energy bodies. These subtle energy bodies, in the attempt to re-align themselves with the physical body, may make the physical body go through a cleansing process as they readjust.

When such yelling is done out of negativity, it can make the etheric body, or the body double, move out of alignment with the physical body. When that happens the body is open to whatever diseases are incubating in it. Each of us has an "etheric body double." Its purpose is to take on an illness before it reaches the physical body. Often, when a person knows how, they can remove an illness from the etheric body double before it gets to the physical body. When a person is ill physically, clearing the etheric body double, along with healing the physical body, can assist with healing.

MN: We've been hearing people talk a lot about the flu. Is there actually a flu virus and can it be transferred from person to person?

J-R: Yes, there is actually a flu virus. The body will create one to match the understanding that there's a flu virus.

MN: You mean if I hear that there's a flu virus then I'll create it?

J-R: You can create a flu virus and you can create a place inside you to receive the flu virus from somebody else. It's a real virus but it wasn't there until people started creating it. In the field of medicine, if I am doing an experiment and I'm looking through a microscope at some virus or cells or some other rarified element, I will influence it by merely looking at it.

MN: So if that scientist sees that for the first time and says, "Oh my God, look at that virus!" and then reports it, the idea just starts growing?

J-R: But a scientist could also look at something and report it with all due accuracy and later be in a different state of consciousness and can't reproduce the experiment. Now in physics there's a classical lab approach to do an experiment in order to get known results. If you don't, you do that experiment over and over until you do get the results you are looking for. You become a scientific physicist who produces mundane, methodical results. The creative experimentation is gone.

MN: That seems a statement about the state of the world!

J-R: We keep reproducing the same old results in order to maintain stability, yet we all say we want newness. But we won't go into the consciousness of adventure that enables us to reach out and get new things. Yet that's what we're all crying out for. We look at somebody and say, "What's new? Tell me something new." Then when a new idea is given we say, "I don't believe it. I don't like it. Something's wrong." It doesn't fit our patterning.

MN: Does counseling help to get to the root of a disease?

**J-R:** If a disease has come out of a psychological misunderstanding then it would really help a person to understand how they created the thought pattern that set up the energy that got into the body. If a person has a good counselor, they can come to the cause/effect basis really fast.

However, a lot of things can clear up just in the process of living. I often can clear up a back problem by getting up and walking around. I can clear up a neck problem by sitting differently. Do you get what I'm saying? It's a simple, mundane approach. I can clear body pains up by leading more with my right foot for a while, instead of my left foot, to rebalance the body.

MN: Is diet important to health?

**J-R:** Yes. If a body is over acid or over alkaline, diet will bring it back into balance. A good acid/alkaline balance is a good place to start for body health. Also, a good approach is to be selective in what you eat rather than too restrictive. It's a very individual thing that has to do with what our body can assimilate. Our desire patterns of eating or our appetites are not as important as what our body can utilize. Once we get over our addictive eating patterns and habits then we can start eating nutritiously. A lot of the body problems that distract us emotionally and mentally can then disappear and we become freer.

MN: It's so simple and practical.

**J-R:** It has to be. It has to be applicable to any human being in any location.

MN: Then, is it just a matter of maintenance or vigilance?

**J-R:** Vigilance is a good word because vigilance is a state of watching. I can elevate my blood pressure by eating potato chips that I love to eat, but they're too salty. I have to question myself as to whether I want elevated blood pressure or whether I want the taste of the potato chips. What I do is I check my blood pressure to see if it's down low enough to know how many potato chips I can eat. (Smiles). So I can have a little bit and get away with it. But I can't be addicted to it because I don't care to have elevated blood pressure.

MN: That's the way I have it worked out with hot fudge sundaes. I can't eat a whole one but I can have a few bites and that's as satisfying to me as eating a whole one.

**J-R:** When we restrict ourselves in our eating, we can then also become obsessive towards the restriction and try to find a way to cheat and get around it. But if we give ourselves the diet of selection, then we can select a little ice cream, or a little bit of fudge later on. We don't sit down and pig out at it until our skin breaks out in repudiation of what we've eaten. Then you're not feeling denied nor are you denying yourself the tastes of life. You've got it in a balanced state, so you can have it.

MN: Throughout history, we have conquered diseases like smallpox, polio, or the bubonic plague. Yet there always seems to be something else that takes its place. Is disease a natural state or is health a natural state?

**J-R:** Although disease appears to be the normal state, the natural state would be health. A human being is a health-seeking, spirit-seeking organism, seeking to expand and grow. That's our nature. Anything that curtails that produces dis-ease.

MN: How does the consciousness of the planet create a bubonic plague or cancer or AIDS, or diseases like that?

**J-R:** Those are all processes of individual disagreement within each person. Many people who get AIDS have given themselves over to something that they have made bigger than them. The thing they've given themselves over to can't fulfill them so they actually are in a state of giving up in the negative sense. When they give up, the immunological system gives up right along with them.

MN: Is that something that we've set up?

**J-R:** We set up everything. There's no way we can blame other people for our own well-being. You're in your body and I'm in mine and we're responsible for them. If you don't exercise those responsibilities, there's no need to blame somebody else for what's going on.

Being in a body, we want to be in control. We want to control what's going to happen so we know there will be a good outcome. We don't want a bad outcome. Even a person who says, "I don't have control," is seeking control through empathy. Control becomes an addiction. It brings us right back to the fear of death. If I knew how I was going to die, and how everything was going to be, I'd be okay because I wouldn't be worrying about a temporary health situation.

MN: Do people contract certain diseases before they incarnate?

J-R: No, we contract lessons. A lot of diseases are needed for our own individual consciousness to grow because it serves a purpose inside of us. When that purpose has been served, then the disease symptoms leave. Then we're in a state of no disease, but I can't call that health. It's just a no-disease state.

MN: So how can people break the cycle of disease?

J-R: I think the most fundamental approach to breaking any cycle is to come back to the consciousness of Self—"to thine own self be true." We work to come to that place. When we find Self we no longer have need or attachment for any other thing. That doesn't mean that we can't respond and enjoy other things, but we're not on a need level where we die emotionally if we don't have that. When we die emotionally, we're shutting off the energy flow. When energy shuts off, disease appears.

MN: Can we, through awakening ourselves, wake up those cells that have been dead and thereby come into a state of better health?

J-R: Absolutely. As you move more into your Self you find less need and greed for the world and then you're no longer a victim to it. When you're not a victim you start to move into a state of health. That doesn't mean that a person can't have an ill state periodically because there may be a need for that—a lesson to be learned. Once it's been learned, we can reach the simple yet profound understanding that we are truly created in God's image, that we truly are an extension of God's essence, and that there is nothing except God. In the fullness of that understanding we enlighten ourselves immediately and the illness that was in the body drops away. It's often called a miraculous healing. This profound, radical understanding takes place inside of a person and it can't be explained to anybody. I can't put words on it.

MN:  What's the prime element for good health?

**J-R:** There would have to be more than one. First of all, good health would be good assimilation, good digestion, good circulation, and good elimination. If all of those aspects are functioning well, we have a state of health by my definition.

MN:  And what would your definition of health be?

**J-R:** Those four things in balance.

MN:  Would that mean more energy in the physical body?

**J-R:** Energy that's usable. A good state of health would be for every thought, a feeling to match it and then move upon it physically to completion. You don't have an excess of anything. There's a balance. In other words, you don't want to have more physical energy than you know what to do with. You don't want to have more thoughts than you can carry out and complete. You don't want to be emotionally distraught or out of balance with more than you can handle. You'd rather have the emotional energy to motivate you to complete physically what you think you need to do.

MN:  It's like the four corners of a square foundation.

**J-R:** Actually it's a triangle. The base is physical, the left side is feeling, and the right side is thought. What you have is a feeling, a thought to match it, and you move on it physically. Now, if you have a thought and a feeling and you can't do anything with it physically, forget it because it will beat you up. If you can't move on it physically, let it go. Or, you could write it down so you can get your thoughts clear. We feel better when we have it off our mind.

MN:  Of the three aspects on the triangle, which one do people most not do?

**J-R:** The physical.

MN:  Does that mean regular exercise or just acting on something we need to do?

**J-R:** Action, putting your body on the line. Faith is a process of mind and emotion, but faith without works is dead. "Works" is physical. The foundation for the understanding is the physical movement.

MN: Where does weight come in?

J-R: Weight, physical body weight, is excess energy fields that you're hanging onto that you don't need. If a time of famine ever appears, the person with a lot of weight is going to last longer than the others. So there's one value to having weight. But weight gets too much negative focus. If we realize that the body weight that we're handling is necessary to us at this time, then we take it in our stride. But when we set up rules and regulations about what our weight should be and it's not matching that ideal, then we distract ourselves from handling our life and we use weight as the thing to beat ourselves up. We're actually avoiding relationships with ourselves and with others. Go to the movie, be with your husband, be with your wife, go talk to your kids, go talk to the teacher about your grades, go talk to your boss about what's happening. Don't avoid the relationship by eating. When we handle our relationships, there's not the need for excess energy, so we don't require more food. Energy from food is utilized differently than the energy involved in relationships. They are different energy fields. When we avoid relationships, those energies get mixed up in the body, our nature becomes confused, and we put on weight. We can tell from looking at the way weight is distributed in the body what the primary issue a person is dealing with inside of them.

MN: What they are holding onto?

J-R: Yes. I often tell people that they carry a lot of excess baggage they don't need. Instead of adding to themselves to find out what's going on, they need to take away what they don't need in order to find out what's going on. When what they don't need has been taken away, what's left is obviously usable to them and they can be free in what they have.

MN: How can I protect myself from a polluted physical environment?

J-R: The best thing to do is to keep a Light consciousness present at all times. It's the best filter there is. Put a shield of Light around you that will filter all the elements coming into you. Bless what you eat and drink, and place the Light with it. Keeping the Light present on all things will be your best protection. When you have a Light attunement, you can put the Light on everything and help transmute it.

MN: Would it be a scary thing for somebody to have a spiritual healing?

J-R: Well it's only scary if it's unknown to the person or if it's shrouded in mysticism. "Greater is he that's in you than he that is in the world." It's a spiritual statement from the Bible. In that, there's nothing to be scared about because we all know inside that we're greater than what we do. The inner part of us is being perfected into God through Christ all the time. All the time. The outer part of us hopes it's being perfected. Now if we give our disease over to a higher form, not as a submission statement, but as a higher gesture of cooperation, where we realize that God knows how to heal us more than we do, we can benefit from this higher state on all of our levels.

MN: How do we do that?

J-R: Prayer.

MN: Just ask?

J-R: Not only just ask, but pray fervently with emotion and depth and fire and conviction and claiming that. Then meditate and allow God to reach into you, tell you, be with you, so you can sense or hear Him. It's called "waiting on the Lord." Another way is contemplation, just looking at the wonder of God, being in awe of a sunset, a flower, a baby, another human being—the attitude of "God did this, it's marvelous!" Watching the surf coming in, listening to birds. There are just so many things we can contemplate where we're in awe of beauty. It's a Zen state, it just is. The other way is spiritual exercises where we leave the body and meet God in the Spirit and become one in the great Spirit with God. That produces great abundance in all of our levels, but mostly spiritually.

MN: So where are we all going?

J-R: To God.

# GLOSSARY

**ACTH** Adrenalcorticotrophic hormone —a hormone secreted by the pituitary gland to stimulate the production of cortisol and other adrenal hormones.

**Adrenaline** *See epinephrine.*

**ANI-HU** A chant used in MSIA. Hu is Sanskrit and is an ancient name for God, and Ani adds the quality of empathy.

**Antioxidants** Substances that inhibit chemical oxidation in the body.

**Astral realm** The psychic, material realm above the physical realm. The realm of the imagination. Intertwines with the physical as a vibratory rate.

**Aura** The electromagnetic energy field that surrounds the human body. Has color and movement.

**Auto-immune disorders** A process where a person's immune system attacks one or more parts of their own body.

**Baruch bashan** (bay-roosh´ bay-shan´) Hebrew words meaning "the blessings already are." The blessings of Spirit exist in the here and now.

**Basic self** Has responsibility for bodily functions; maintains habits and the psychic centers of the physical body. Also known as the lower self. Handles prayers from the physical to the high self. See also conscious self and high self.

**Beloved** The Soul; the God within.

**Chakra** A psychic center of the body.

**Christ Consciousness** A universal consciousness of pure Spirit. Exists within each person through the Soul.

**Conscious self** The self that makes conscious choices. It is the "captain of the ship" in that it can override both the basic self and the high self. The self that comes in as a tabula rasa. See also basic self and high self.

**Cortisol** Also known as hydrocortisone, is a corticosteroid hormone or glucocorticoid produced by the zona fasciculata of the adrenal cortex, which is one of the two parts of the adrenal gland. It is released in response to stress, or to a low level of blood glucocorticoids.

**CRF** Corticotrophin releasing factor—the hormone secreted by the hypothalamus that directs the pituitary to create adrenal corticotrophic hormones (ACTH). CRF is the major regulator of the production of cortisol.

**Crown Chakra** The psychic center at the top of the head.

**Discourses** See *Soul Awareness Discourses.*

**Endocrine glands** Glands that secrete hormones directly into the bloodstream, influencing metabolism and other body processes. The endocrine glands include the hypothalamus, pituitary, thyroid, parathyroid, adrenals, thymus, pineal, and gonads (ovaries and testicles).

**Epinephrine** A hormone secreted by the adrenal glands especially in conditions of stress, increasing rates of blood circulation, breathing, carbohydrate metabolism, and preparing muscles for exertion. Also called adrenaline.

**Etheric realm** The psychic, material realm above the mental realm and below the Soul realm. Equated with the unconscious or subconscious level. Sometimes known as the esoteric realm.

**False self** Can be thought of as the ego, the individualized personality that incorrectly perceives itself to be fundamentally separated from others and God.

**Glucocorticoids** Steroids secreted by the adrenal cortex. The name glucocorticoid (glucose + cortex + steroid) derives from their role in the regulation of the metabolism of glucose (blood sugar), their synthesis in the adrenal cortex, and their steroidal structure. They are part of the feedback mechanism in the immune system that turns immune activity (inflammation) down. The most common glucocorticoid is cortisol.

**Gluconeogenesis** One of the two main mechanisms the body uses to keep blood glucose levels from dropping too low (hypoglycemia) by converting fatty acids or amino acids into glucose.

**High self** The self that functions as one's spiritual guardian, directing the conscious self towards those experiences that are for one's greatest spiritual progression. Has knowledge of the destiny pattern agreed upon before embodiment. *See also basic self, conscious self, and Karmic Board.*

**Holy Spirit** The positive energy of Light and Sound that comes from the Supreme God. The life force that sustains everything in all creation. Often uses the magnetic Light through which to work on the psychic, material realms. Works only for the highest good. Is the third part of the Trinity or Godhead.

**Homeostasis** The tendency of a healthy body towards a stable equilibrium of body mechanisms and processes.

**HU** A "tone," or sound, that is an ancient name of the Supreme God.

**Hypothalamus** An endocrine gland situated in the brain that regulates most of the functions of the endocrine system and many other automatic functions of the body.

**Inflammation** A reaction in the body to injury or infection that involves redness, swelling, heat, and sometimes pain and loss of function.

**Initiation** In MSIA, the process of being connected to the Sound Current of God.

**Initiation tone** In MSIA, spiritually charged words given to an initiate in a Sound Current initiation. The name of the Lord of the realm into which the person is being initiated.

**Inner levels/realms** The astral, causal, mental, etheric, and Soul realms that exist within a person's consciousness. See also *outer levels/realms.*

**Insulin resistance** The lack of response of cells to the presence of insulin.

**Karma** The law of cause and effect: as you sow, so shall you reap. The responsibility of each person for his or her actions. The law that directs and sometimes dominates a being's physical existence.

**Karmic Board** A group of nonphysical spiritual masters who meet with a being before embodiment to assist in the planning of that being's spiritual journey on Earth. The Mystical Traveler has a function in this group.

**Light** The energy of Spirit that pervades all realms of existence. Also refers to the Light of the Holy Spirit.

**Light, magnetic** The Light of God that functions in the psychic, material realms. Not as high as the Light of the Holy Spirit, and does not necessarily function for the highest good. See also Light and Holy Spirit.

**Line of the Travelers** The line of spiritual energy extending from the Mystical Traveler Consciousness, in which the Mystical Traveler's students function.

**Mental realm** The psychic, material realm above the causal realm and below the etheric realm. Relates to the universal mind.

**Movement of Spiritual Inner Awareness (MSIA)** An organization whose major focus is to bring people into an awareness of Soul Transcendence. John-Roger is the founder.

**Mystical Traveler Consciousness** An energy from the highest source of Light and Sound whose spiritual directive on Earth is awakening people to the awareness of the Soul. This consciousness always exists on the planet through a physical form.

**Negative realms** See *psychic, material realms*.

**Outer levels/realms** The astral, causal, mental, etheric, and Soul realms above the Soul realm also exist outside a person's consciousness, but in a greater way. See also *inner levels/realms*.

**Peace Theological Seminary and College of Philosophy (PTS)** A private, non-denominational institution presenting the spiritual teachings of MSIA.

**Physical realm** The earth. The psychic, material realm in which a being lives with a physical body.

**Pituitary gland** A major endocrine gland that is pea-sized and attached to the base of the brain. It is important in controlling growth and development and the functioning of the other endocrine glands.

**Positive realms** The Soul realm and the 27 levels above the Soul realm. See also *psychic, material realms*.

**Psychic, material realms** The five lower, negative realms; namely, the physical, astral, causal, mental, and etheric realms. See also *positive realms*.

**Seeding** A form of prayer to God for something that one wants to manifest in the world. It is done by placing a "seed" with (giving an amount of money to) the source of one's spiritual teachings.

**S.e.'s** See *spiritual exercises*.

**Soul** The extension of God individualized within each human being. The basic element of human existence, forever connected to God. The indwelling Christ, the God within.

**Soul Awareness Discourses** Booklets that students in MSIA read monthly as their spiritual study, for individual, private and personal use only. They are an important part of the Traveler's teachings on the physical level.

**Soul consciousness** A positive state of being. Once a person is established in Soul consciousness, he or she need no longer be bound or influenced by the lower levels of Light.

**Soul realm** The realm above the etheric realm. The first of the positive realms and the true home of the Soul. The first level where the Soul is consciously aware of its true nature, its pure beingness, its oneness with God.

**Soul transcendence** The process of moving the consciousness beyond the psychic, material realms and into the Soul realm and beyond.

**Soul travel** Traveling in Spirit to realms of consciousness other than the physical realm.

Sometimes known as out-of-body experiences. This can be done in one's own inner realms or in the outer realms, the higher spiritual realms. See also *inner levels/realms and outer levels/realms*.

**Sound Current** The audible energy that flows from God through all realms. The spiritual energy on which a person returns to the heart of God.

**Spirit** The essence of creation. Infinite and eternal.

**Spiritual exercises (s.e.'s)** Chanting the HU, the ANI-HU, or one's initiation tone. An active technique of bypassing the mind and emotions by using a spiritual tone to connect to the Sound Current. Assists a person in breaking through the illusions of the lower levels and eventually moving into Soul consciousness. See also *initiation tone*.

**Spiritual eye** The area in the center of the head, back from the center of the forehead. Used to see inwardly. Also called the third eye.

**Tithing** The spiritual practice of giving 10 percent of one's increase to God by giving it to the source of one's spiritual teachings.

**Universal Mind** Located at the highest part of the etheric realm, at the division between the negative and positive realms. Gets its energy from the mental realm. The source of the individual mind.

# BIBLIOGRAPHY

Readers who are seeking more scientific depth relating to the section *Applying the Principles*, may find the following books a good place to start:

*ON STRESS:*

**Adrenal Fatigue: The 21st Century Stress Syndrome**
by James L. Wilson, N.D., D.C., Ph.D., *Smart Publications*;
(January 25, 2002)

**Why Zebras Don't Get Ulcers** by Robert M. Sapolsky,
*Holt Paperbacks; 3rd edition* (August 26, 2004)

*ON CELLS:*

**How We Live and Why We Die: The Secret Lives of Cells**
by Lewis Wolpert, *Faber and Faber*; (April 1, 2010)

*ON ACID/ALKALINE BALANCE:*

**The Chemistry of Success: Six Secrets of Peak Performance**
by Susan M. Lark, M.D. and James A. Richards, M.B.A., *Bay Books;*
*First Edition* (2000)

## Forgiveness
The Key to the Kingdom

Forgiveness is the key factor in personal liberation and spiritual progression. This book presents profound insights into forgiveness and the resulting personal joy and freedom. God's business is forgiving. This book provides encouragement and techniques for making it our business as well.

*Softbound Book* ISBN #9780914829621, **$12.95**

## Momentum: Letting Love Lead
Simple Practices for Spiritual Living
*(with Paul Kaye, D.S.S.)*

As much as we might like to have the important areas of our lives - Relationships, Health, Finances and Career—all settled and humming along, the reality for most of us is that there is always something out of balance, often causing stress and distress. Rather than resisting or regretting imbalance, this book shows that there is an inherent wisdom in imbalance. Where there is imbalance, there is movement, and that movement "gives rise to a dynamic, engaging life that is full of learning, creativity, and growth."

We can discover—in the very areas where we experience most of our problems and challenges—the greatest movement and the greatest opportunity for change.

The approach is not to try harder at making life work. Life already works. The big key is to bring loving into it. This book is about being loving in the moment. It is a course in loving.

*Hardbound book* ISBN #9781893020184, **$19.95**

## The Rest of Your Life
Finding Repose in the Beloved
*(with Paul Kaye, D.S.S.)*

What if you discovered that rest is less an action and more an attitude? That you can gain all the inner and outer benefits of rest as you move through each day, no matter how busy you are? Here is the good news: It's true, and you can. If you ever told yourself you could do with a good rest, this book will serve you well. Starting now, for the rest of your life.

*Softbound book* ISBN #9781893020436, **$16.95**

*The following books and audio materials can support you in learning more about the ideas presented in "Living the Spiritual Principles of Health and Well-Being."*

*They can be ordered through the Movement of Spiritual Inner Awareness at: (323) 737-4055, www.msia.org, order@msia.org*

## When Are You Coming Home?

A Personal Guide to Soul Transcendence

*(with Pauli Sanderson, D.S.S.)*

An intimate account of spiritual awakening that contains the elements of an adventure story. How did John-Roger attain the awareness of who he truly is? He approached life like a scientist in a laboratory. He found methods for integrating the sacred with the mundane, the practical with the mystical. He noted what worked and what didn't. Along with some fascinating stories, you will find in this book many practical keys for making your own life work better, for attuning to the source of wisdom that is always within you, and for making every day propel you further on your exciting adventure home. Includes a guided meditation by John-Roger on CD *Inner Journey Through Spirit Realms*.

*Hardbound book*   ISBN#9781893020238, **$19.95**

## What's It Like Being You?

*(with Paul Kaye, D.S.S.)*

What would happen if you stopped doing what you thought you were supposed to be doing and started being who you are? The sequel to their previous book together, *Momentum – Letting Love Lead*, this book features exercises, meditations and narrative to deepen and explore who you really are as well as a new CD release *Meditation for Alignment with the True Self.*

*Softbound book*   ISBN#9781893020252, **$14.95**

## Spiritual Warrior:

The Art of Spiritual Living

Full of wisdom, humor, common sense, and hands-on tools for spiritual living, this book offers practical tips to take charge of our lives and create greater health, happiness, abundance, and loving. Becoming a spiritual warrior has nothing to do with violence. It is about using the positive qualities of the spiritual warrior—intention, ruthlessness, and impeccability—to counter negative personal habits and destructive relationships, especially when you are confronted with great adversity.

*Softbound book*   ISBN#9781893020481, **$14.95**

## The Tao of Spirit

This beautifully designed collection of writings is intended to free you from outer worldly distractions and guide your return to the stillness within. The Tao of Spirit can provide daily inspirations and new approaches on how to handle stress and frustration. What a wonderful way to start or to end the day—remembering to let go of your day-to-day problems and be refreshed in the source at the center of your existence. Many people use this book in preparation for meditation or prayer.

*Hardbound book*   ISBN#9780914829331, **$15**

## Inner Worlds of Meditation

In this self-help guide to meditation, meditation practices are transformed into valuable and practical resources for exploring the spiritual realms and dealing with life more effectively. Included are a variety of meditations that can be used for gaining spiritual awareness, achieving greater relaxation, balancing the emotions, and increasing energy.

*Softbound Book*   ISBN#9780914829454, **$11.95**
*3-CD packet* #9780914829645, **$30**

*John-Roger's books are available in bookstores everywhere or at www. mandevillepress.org*

## Loving Each Day for Peacemakers:
Choosing Peace Everyday

Peace? It's a noble idea, yet a seemingly elusive reality. Peace between nations is built upon peace between individuals, and peace between individuals depends upon peace within each person. Making peace more than just a theory or idea, *Loving Each Day for Peacemakers* guides readers to their own solutions for experiencing peace.

*Hardbound book*   ISBN#9781893020146, **$12**

## Psychic Protection

In this book, John-Roger describes some of the invisible levels: the power of thoughts, the unconscious, elemental energies, and magic. More important, he discusses how to protect yourself from negativity that can be part of those levels. As you practice the simple techniques in this book, you can create a greater sense of well-being in and around you.

*Softbound Book*   ISBN#9780914829690, **$6.95**

## Health from the Inside Out

The seminars in this set of 3 CDs outline how to use the energy of the body, starting at the cell level, to create better health. They include insights into and methods for overcoming the cycle of overeating. There is a description of the power of your thoughts and how to use this power for better health, as well as how to connect with the Supreme Source to promote healing and vitality. *"This whole world boils down to one word—energy—and it's used either for you or against you."* —John-Roger.

*The packet includes:*

- Adapting Toward Health or Adopting Dis-ease
- Are You Stuffing Your Expression?
- Are You Unconsciously Depleting Your Energy?
- Awakening Beyond Body Consciousness
- The Body Balance Meditation

*3-CD packet* #3909-CD, **$25**
*Downloadable* #3909-MP3, **$17.50**

## Health Is Loving Who You Really Are

In this seminar, John-Roger shows how we corrupt the life-sustaining energy of love with anger, rejection, blame, etc.—those experiences which lead to our dis-ease. He describes how these negative energies (and negative habits) get into the body and what they do once they've found a home there.

John-Roger doesn't leave us there, though; he says: "If you could truly flush your system with loving energy…get the system clean… you'd be in health and it would radiate out from you as life-giving energy." In this important seminar, he shows us how.

*CD* #7970-CD, **$10**
*DVD* #7970-DVD, **$20**
*Downloadable* #7970-MP3, **$8**

## Are You Available to Yourself?

Health, wealth, happiness, abundance, and riches are our heritage in this life. John-Roger reminds us that everything is available to us if we are available to ourselves and the spiritual life-force within us all.

*CD* #7238-CD, **$10**
*Downloadable* #7238-MP3, **$8**

## Observation, The Key to Letting Go

In order to accept what is, we need to observe, like a scientist. "Observation," John-Roger says, "is the key to letting go and letting God." In observation, we are not getting involved with our emotions or bringing preconceived assumptions to the situation. Learning how to practice these principles more effectively can have tangible and profound benefits for bringing greater balance and happiness into our lives.

*CD* #1552-CD, **$10**
*Downloadable* #1552-MP3, **$8**

*To order audio or video materials, contact MSIA at (323) 737-4055, order@msia.org, or simply visit the online store at www.msia.org*

## Getting More Spirit Through Breathing

This is a humorous and information-packed seminar in which John-Roger reminds us that if we want to figure out our first priority, all we need to do is hold our breath as long as we can. All other considerations fall away until we can take in the next breath! J-R gives an excellent technique for expanding our lungs and getting more air in as we breathe. You will learn how to bring more Spirit into you, and more Spirit equates to better health.

*CD* #7653-CD, **$10**
*DVD* #7653-DVD, **$20**

# LIVING IN GRACE

Forgiveness is one of the major keys for living in grace. Forgiveness opens the door to greater inner freedom and an awareness of the grace that is always awaiting us.

This best selling four CD set of talks, which includes a meditation, and an innerphasing (a tool for changing unconscious habits), is designed to guide you into a greater experience of Spirit and of remembering who you truly are.

*To order audio or video materials, contact MSIA at (323) 737-4055, order@msia.org, or simply visit the online store at www.msia.org*

### Consciousness of Grace
*Grace is God's dispensation that allows those things which have been out of balance in your life to be balanced instantly. This seminar offers keys for lifting yourself into the consciousness of grace.*

### Are You Living Under Law or Grace?
*An enlightening look at how to live your daily life in the grace that is always available. Lists 24 qualities of grace - and their opposites, "the law."*

### Meditation on Forgiveness
*A tender meditation in which you are gently guided into the loving of the Christ where all things can be forgiven and truly healed.*

### Forgiveness Innerphasing
*Leads you through ten levels of consciousness into the "basic self," bringing forgiveness, healing, and loving to each level.*

### Free-Form Writing
*Detailed instructions for this technique, which assists you in clearing unconscious blocks to Spirit. Also includes soothing background music which supports the process of releasing.*

### Meditation for Peace
*A meditative journey that calls you forward into the spirit of peace. Assists you in finding more loving, acceptance, and healing through forgiveness and remembering who you really are.*

*4-CD packet #3903-CD,* **$35**
*Downloadable #3903-MP3,* **$24.50**

# SOUL AWARENESS DISCOURSES
## A COURSE IN SOUL TRANSCENDENCE

Soul Awareness Discourses are designed to teach Soul Transcendence, which is becoming aware of yourself as a Soul and as one with God, not as a theory, but as a living reality. They are for people who want a consistent, time-proven approach to their spiritual unfoldment.

A set of Soul Awareness Discourses consists of 12 booklets, one to study and contemplate each month of the year. As you read each Discourse, you can activate an awareness of your Divine essence and deepen your relationship with God.

Spiritual in essence, Discourses are compatible with religious beliefs you might hold. In fact, most people find that Discourses support the experience of whatever path, philosophy, or religion (if any) they choose to follow. Simply put, Discourses are about eternal truths and the wisdom of the heart.

The first year of Discourses addresses topics ranging from creating success in the world to working hand-in-hand with Spirit.

A yearly set of Discourses is regularly $100. MSIA is offering the first year of Discourses at an introductory price of $50. Discourses come with a full, no-questions-asked, money-back guarantee. If at any time you decide this course of study is not right for you, simply return it, and you will promptly receive a full refund.

*To order Discourses, contact the Movement of Spiritual Inner Awareness at (323) 737-4055, order@msia. org or visit the online store at www.msia.org*

# ABOUT THE AUTHORS

## John-Roger, D.S.S.

A teacher and lecturer of international stature, John-Roger is an inspiration in the lives of many people around the world. For over four decades, his wisdom, humor, common sense and love have helped people to discover the Spirit within themselves and find health, peace, and prosperity.

*For more information about John-Roger, you may also visit: www.john-roger.org*

With two co-authored books on the *New York Times* Bestseller List to his credit, and more than four dozen self-help books and audio albums, John-Roger offers extraordinary insights on a wide range of topics. He is the founder and spiritual adviser of the non-denominational Church of the Movement of Spiritual Inner Awareness (MSIA), which focuses on Soul Transcendence; founder, first president, and now chancellor of the University of Santa Monica; founder and chancellor of Peace Theological Seminary and College of Philosophy; founder and chairman of the board of Insight Seminars; founder and spiritual adviser of the Institute for Individual and World Peace; and founder of The Heartfelt Foundation.

John-Roger has given over 6,000 lectures and seminars worldwide, many of which are televised nationally on his cable program, "*That Which Is*," through the Network of Wisdoms. He has appeared on numerous radio and television shows and has been a featured guest on "*Larry King Live*." He also co-wrote and co-produced the movie *Spiritual Warriors* (www.**spiritualwarriors**.com).

An educator and minister by profession, John-Roger continues to transform lives by educating people in the wisdom of the spiritual heart.

## Paul Kaye, D.S.S.

Paul Kaye has been a dedicated student of spiritual thought and practices since his youth in England. His explorations have taken him into Yoga, Zen, and the spiritual foundations of movement and the martial arts.

Paul's interests include the philosophies of such poets and teachers as Lao Tzu, Rumi and Kabir and the esoteric teachings of Jesus Christ. Paul has designed workshops on the practical application of spiritual principles and presented them worldwide. Paul is a unique and remarkable presence. He brings an abundance of lightheartedness into whatever he does, and his presentations are inspiring, practical, and filled with a wonderful sense of humor and wisdom.

For over 30 years he has studied with renowned educator and author John-Roger and he is president of the Church of the Movement of Spiritual Inner Awareness (MSIA), an ecumenical, non-denominational church. Paul is an ordained minister and has a doctorate in spiritual science.

*For author interviews and speaking engagements please contact Angel Harper at 3500 West Adams Blvd. Los Angeles, CA 90018 (323) 737-4055 x1180 Angel@ mandevillepress.org*

# ACKNOWLEDGMENTS AND THANKS

A conversation at a friend's birthday party in 2002 started Mark Holmes, O.M.D., and I (Paul Kaye) thinking about the many resources on achieving greater health and well-being that we have at our disposal thanks to John-Roger's teachings, and how under utilized these resources were. In subsequent meetings over several weeks, we crafted an eight-week class through Peace Theological Seminary and College of Philosophy called *The Spiritual Principles of Health and Well-Being*. The key elements of that class form the basis of this book. Philip Barr, M.D., and Diane Botticelli assisted us in facilitating and shaping the class.

Philip and Diane have continued to give their invaluable input and assisted greatly in reviewing and offering their suggestions on the more technical aspects of this book.

Additional thanks go to Barbara Wieland whose search for material in the John-Roger Library and Archives yielded many of the J-R gems you'll find in this book. Nancy O'Leary and Carrie Hopkins were a delight to work with, and their copy-editing brings a greater lucidity to the material. Virginia Rose volunteered her expert eyes in proofreading the completed manuscript. And Bambi Lyn Scott cast her eye over the final draft and managed to improve it even more.

Vincent Dupont shared his expertise and perspective to help shape the content. And Shelley Noble's design put the finishing touches to a book that we hope will be a useful resource for many years to come.

Heartfelt thanks to you all.

We welcome your comments and questions.

## Mandeville Press

P.O. Box 513935
Los Angeles, CA 90051-1935
(323) 737-4055

jrbooks@**mandeville**press.org

www.**mandeville**press.org